WITHDRAWN

BY BOB HARPER

Skinny Habits

Skinny Meals

Jumpstart to Skinny

The Skinny Rules

Are You Ready!

SKINNY HABITS

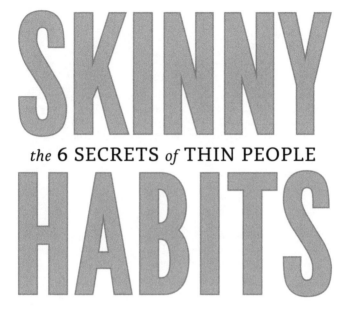

SKINNY HABITS

the **6** SECRETS *of* THIN PEOPLE

BOB HARPER

with **Greg Critser**

BALLANTINE BOOKS

NEW YORK

No book can replace the diagnostic expertise and medical advice of a trusted physician. Please be certain to consult with your doctor before making any decisions that affect your health or extreme changes in your diet, particularly if you suffer from any medical condition or have any symptom that may require treatment.

Some names and identifying details have been changed.

Published in the United States by Ballantine Books, an imprint of Random House, a division of Penguin Random House LLC, New York.

BALLANTINE and the HOUSE colophon are registered trademarks of Penguin Random House LLC.

LIBRARY OF CONGRESS CATALOGING-IN-PUBLICATION DATA
Harper, Bob.
Skinny habits : the 6 secrets of thin people / Bob Harper ;
Greg Critser.
pages cm.
Includes bibliographical references and index.
ISBN 978-0-8041-7890-7
eBook ISBN 978-0-8041-7891-4
1. Weight loss. 2. Weight loss—Psychological aspects.
I. Critser, Greg. II. Title.
RM222.2.H2447 2015
613.2'5—dc23 2015000507

Yoga pose illustrations by Neal Rohrer

Printed in the United States of America on acid-free paper

www.ballantinebooks.com

2 4 6 8 9 7 5 3 1

First Edition

Book design by Casey Hampton

This book is dedicated to my godchildren,
Audrey Colette and Miles Maximus Marantette Murphy,
aka Coco and Miles. I love you both so much.
You have filled a hole in my heart that I didn't know
I had until I met you both. You make me laugh and
you are the coolest people I know. BFFs for life!

CONTENTS

Introduction: The Secrets of Skinny   xi

1. The Skinny Mindset   3

2. The Skinny Brain   11

3. Habit 1: Make Contingency Plans   23

4. Habit 2: Consciously Push Back   43

5. Habit 3: Reengineer Your Environment   67

6. Habit 4: Challenge Yourself   89

7. Habit 5: Rest for Success   103

8. Habit 6: Dress for Thin   131

Skinny Is as Skinny Does   149

Acknowledgments   151

Notes   153

Index   159

The Skinny Habits Recap   173

The Skinny Rules Recap   175

THE SECRETS OF SKINNY

As perhaps you know, for more than ten years I have worked with obese people on NBC's *The Biggest Loser,* training and coaching them on how to lose weight for weekly competitive weigh-ins; on the show, the person who loses the highest percentage of body fat wins. For even longer than that—more than twenty-five years in all—I have trained private clients who often had less to lose than the *TBL* contestants, but pounds they needed to shed nonetheless. In other words, I witness—up close—the lives of people trying to lose weight every single day.

I coach all these people to eat better (and less) and work out efficiently (and more), and I never stop preaching my "twenty nonnegotiable rules for getting to thin," the nutritional dos and don'ts that I detailed in my 2012 book, *The*

Skinny Rules. Those twenty rules really work (they are reprinted at the back of this book so you can refresh your memory), and I've seen countless inspiring transformations when people stick to them. Amazing weight loss, proud smiles, new wardrobes. Amazing health improvements, happy doctors and spouses, a new lease on life!

What's the key phrase there? *When people stick to them!* Because of course people start off great and lose some weight, but then they partly revert to their old eating and nonexercising patterns and, no surprise, their weight loss plateaus well shy of the number on the scale they were aiming for. Unfortunately, too many people revert to their old ways completely and over time gain back even more than they'd lost.

It usually starts with some small slipup (say, you eat one more brownie than you'd set as your limit), which leads to irrational and unproductive shame (*I'm never going to lose this weight because I'm weak, so what's the point of even trying?*) and you binge (an entire "splurge week"!), which sets you off on a course to increasingly unhealthy behavior and yet more shame. This slip-shame-binge cycle is the bane of every dieter's existence.

The fact that you're reading this book tells me you'd like the madness to stop. You want to lose weight once and for all. And then you'd really, really like to stop worrying about it! Wouldn't it be nice to move on to other concerns?

You've come to the right place. Because in all my time of coaching and training and encouraging and taking notes, I've figured out what differentiates the people who stick to the plan from those who don't. In other words, I've figured out what differentiates *them* from *you*. And I know how to make you one of *them*! The best news yet? You don't have to have a personal trainer or coach, a personal chef or nutritionist to master these patterns. What we're talking about in this book is *not* what you put in your mouth and how often you get off the couch and into the gym.

Boiled down, what separates the consistently healthy and slim from the chronically overweight are six key thought patterns and behaviors: six habits. By the time you turn the last page in this book, you're going to understand what I understand, see what I see, and be able to begin making the small mental and physical changes needed to turn things around for you.

For good.

SKINNY THOUGHTS, SKINNY ACTIONS

A slipup is an action: you eat that darn brownie. And another.

Shame is a mindset. You berate yourself for your "weak" behavior; you feel pessimistic about ever being the kind of person who can resist fattening food or who can get herself to exercise regularly.

And so you binge and/or go back to your unhealthy behavior. More destructive action.

Slip-shame-binge is an action-thought-action cycle, right?

The six habits you'll learn in this book will break that

terrible cycle for good. Some are habits of the mind, some are physical things you do. Habits 1 and 2 focus on the psychological portion of the cycle, toughening you up mentally to fight your worst tendencies; Habits 3–6 get you out of your head and into things you can touch and change and undertake immediately.

So, what do healthy and slim people know and do that you don't? Here's a quick overview to get you excited:

1. *They plan:* To avoid unhealthy eating, encourage exercise, resist temptation, and guard against that first slip, healthy and thin people create their own internal scripts for dealing with difficult but unavoidable situations.

2. *They push back:* Using simple, proven psychological techniques, they have developed and maintained the mental muscle to deal with setbacks (aka the cascading shame from that inevitable slip!).

3. *They reengineer their environment:* Successful weight maintainers have rigged their world to accentuate the people, places, and things that support their goals, and they deemphasize (or eliminate) those that don't.

4. *They challenge themselves:* Boredom is the gateway to overeating and sitting around like a lump on your couch. Having a hobby or a mission keeps the mind engaged and excited about something other than the monotony of daily responsibilities.

5. *They rest:* You can be engaged, excited, focused, and energized only if you are rested. Thin and healthy people protect their sleep and relaxation, understanding the connection between rest and weight control.

6. *They dress for thinness:* Thin and healthy people dress like they have something to show, not hide. Even if they aren't aware of the fascinating science underlying their choices, they enjoy the psychological and physiological benefits of what's in their wardrobe (and what's not).

Here's what I want you to get your head around before you turn the page: *you are not at the mercy of your current bad habits.* You can replace your poor habits with healthy ones—the six above—faster than you might think. As you'll learn in Chapter 1, changing/replacing a bad habit with a good one takes practice, but that's why each habit has "Habit Homework" at the end of the chapter—ideas for ways you can start making new routines and laying down new neural pathways right away.

When you plan for challenges and situations—when you think about how you want to behave in situations that have always broken your resolve in the past—you can create new go-to behaviors. When you push back against automatic and irrational thoughts, you train your brain to go to a happier place instead of a negative and unproductive one. When you set up your environment to support your goals, you reach them. When you challenge yourself, and yet also rest, you give your brain the one-two punch it needs to stay the course. When you dress for thinness, you get there.

Let's get started!

SKINNY HABITS

one

THE SKINNY MINDSET

This isn't your first rodeo. I know that you know a thing or two about the simple math of energy in and energy out (i.e., you've got to burn more energy through movement than you put in through your mouth in the form of food), and you've studied up a bit on nutrition (a whole lot less processed food, a whole lot more vegetables). You probably have a handle on what you need to do to manipulate your metabolism to burn more fat. And I'm guessing you have experienced firsthand the way your body sometimes reacts to your attempted manipulations: if it thinks that you're going through a drought or famine, it does its best to *store* fat to protect you. Unfair, but true.

The details of what to put in your mouth and how much to exercise are, of course, super important when it comes to weight loss and weight maintenance, and I want you to learn as much as you can about nutrients and calories and the importance of timing when it comes to eating. Again, I encourage you to read *The Skinny Rules* for the facts and principles that will put you on a path to a much healthier weight. And I encourage you to cook more for yourself and to try new and weight-friendly recipes. I've got a book for that too: *Skinny Meals.*

But then you've got to follow through on your intentions to cook and eat better, to listen to your body, and to stop eating when you are full! Because that's what skinny people have the willpower to do, right?

But what is willpower? People who don't struggle with their weight seem to have self-control in spades, so much so that it seems natural, effortless. You seem to lack it; conjuring willpower and using it takes a megadose of conscious effort, effort you just don't have in you.

To my trained eye, willpower is all about mindset. More specifically, a "skinny mindset." And there's good science to prove that I'm on to something.

MIND OVER MATTER?

Your mindset is your *outlook on life,* your underlying attitudes, biases, and assumptions about how the world works and your place in it; it's a disposition shaped by years of experiences and countless influences. What you were exposed to as a child contributes to your present-day mindset: your parents' and friends' attitudes, their politics, their health, their moods, their work ethic. And what you deal with every day shapes it as well: your job, your day-to-day stress level, and the health and mood of the person you're dating or living with (yes, as you'll learn in Chapter 5, who you hang out with is more important than you might think!).

People with what's called a *fixed* mindset believe that strengths and capabilities are pretty much out of individual control. Instead, they believe that capabilities are either *innate* (you're born with them) or attributable to *external* influences and triggers (something someone else does to or for them, something they buy, what they eat or drink).

Those with a *growth* mindset believe that abilities are not finite and also not dependent on an external event or influence; instead, they believe that individual effort can expand and improve talents or capabilities on its own. You can have fixed mindsets about some things and growth mindsets about others. It all depends on what you've been conditioned to believe and in what context.

An example: people with a fixed mindset about their abilities in math believe that their ease with math is something that they were born with, something perhaps they inherited from their math-genius father or mother. Or they believe that being good at math is all about having the right teacher, textbook, or tutoring—it's about someone or something else stepping in to help make you better.

By contrast, people with a growth mindset believe that individual practice and effort can bolster their math skill. They believe that they aren't at the mercy of their family's math lameness or their own perceived limits.

It all comes down to this: Does it matter *what you believe about willpower itself?* Does that belief affect your ability to persevere when the going gets tough?

Consider the work of Carol Dweck, a professor of psychology at Stanford University, and the genius who coined the phrases *fixed mindset* and *growth mindset*.

Before Professor Dweck challenged it, the general assumption was that the body needed extra fuel to boost self-control (willpower), the classic example being the snack— a chocolate bar or cookie (some form of glucose)—in the late afternoon when you're just "so tired." The logic was that mental tasks (like work!) deplete your energy, but a shot of glucose boosts it. I'm betting this is an assumption you've made yourself—after all, it's a great rationalization for that afternoon sugar hit! It's also a great excuse for not being able to control your actions: you can argue that your body is telling you to eat that donut and you are helpless to really push back.

But Dweck didn't buy it. She could see that the body is nothing if not a powerful energy-conscious computer, able to maintain physiological balance so long as it's not being put under great stress (like illness or famine or drought). So she wondered why such an intricate and powerful contraption like the body wouldn't adjust itself—releasing stored glucose from the liver, say—rather than depending on external sources (like a chocolate bar!) when energy or focus starts to wane. She wondered if something psychological, like belief—what she came to call "mindset"—mattered. To test her hunch, she designed a series of ingenious experiments.

First, she used a questionnaire to get a handle on what a large group of people (sixty) felt about willpower. Based on those results, she found that her subjects fell into two groups.

One group consisted of people whose answers showed they felt there's only so much willpower at any individual's command at any given time, and when it's depleted, you lose the self-control you need for any effortful task: exercising, resisting a donut, paying attention—you name it. Obviously, this was the "fixed mindset" crowd.

In contrast, the other group believed that willpower was something dynamic, renewable, plentiful—something you can generate on your own through awareness, hard work, and confidence. These people had a "growth mindset" about willpower.

She hadn't asked these people anything that would suggest she was testing their belief in the glucose–self-control theory, but that's what she was trying to do.

Now it got interesting. Professor Dweck put these people through a series of tests that demanded strenuous mental concentration—crossing out every other *e* in a text, or identifying complex color-shape combinations. Sticking with the challenge took focus and self-control. About halfway through the challenge, she gave both groups a sugary snack (lemonade). What she found was surprising, arguably revolutionary. Writing in a recent article, she noted that "only people who view willpower as limited and easily depleted exhibited improved self-control after sugar consumption. In contrast, people who view willpower as plentiful showed no benefits from glucose—*they exhibited high levels of self-control performance with or without sugar boosts.*"

The italics are mine, and I hope you can see why! The mere *belief* that willpower is limited sensitizes people to bodily cues for fuel—that devilish afternoon snack!—and *that makes them dependent on glucose boosts for high self-control.* In contrast, as Dweck explained, "People who didn't think willpower was limited didn't show a depletion effect after a strenuous task and didn't need sugar to keep going strong. Those people may feel fatigued, but they don't think that means they can't work hard. Our findings suggest that what has been viewed as a basic biological process is really a product of people's beliefs."

A basic biological process is really a product of people's beliefs? Amazing!

You might relate to an even more pointed explanation—one that accounts for a lot of things that happen during weight loss and control. "When you have a limited theory of willpower," Professor Dweck said, "you're constantly on alert, constantly monitoring yourself. 'Am I tired? Am I hungry? Do I need a break? How am I feeling?' And at the first sign that something is flagging, you think, I need a rest or a boost."

Which pretty well sums up the major hurdle of dieters everywhere: if you believe that you need certain *external* things to help you exercise self-control (or that you need certain kinds of foods to help you stay focused, calories be damned), you will not really believe it's possible to override your body's biology. So . . . believe! When it comes to will-power, it really matters!

Now comes the burning question: What does it take to change your mindset? To use the earlier math example, it turns out you can change a kid's view of his or her math ability by regularly and repeatedly talking about math abil-ity as something that is built up through practice and effort instead of something you're born with (and praising the ef-fort that goes into getting those improved grades). And if you're a sports fan, you know that an athlete's repeated and practiced visualization of an improved game is a key com-ponent of making that visualization a reality.

Repeated practice? Yes, we're talking about habits! After all, the outward manifestation of your mindset is your be-havior, the things you do and the way you carry yourself in the world. Your automatic, default behaviors. But also your consciously cultivated routines. How about turning your consciously cultivated routines *into* automatic, default be-haviors? As I said in the introduction, wouldn't it be nice to get to that point and live the rest of your life without con-stantly having to think about creating and maintaining skinny-fying habits? Yes, it would. Read on!

two

THE SKINNY BRAIN

Y

ou've got your head around the need to change your mindset, right? You now understand the faulty logic in your past assumptions about willpower? Instead of shrugging and accepting that you don't have as much willpower as the skinny person next door, you're now going to believe in your own capacity for it, right? Excellent. Glad to have you on board, because forming the six new Skinny Habits is going to take some of that willpower, some of that belief energy!

Maybe you're anxious to just skip ahead and get on with the important business of learning your new Skinny Habits already. I don't blame you and I'm happy for your enthusiasm, quite frankly! You can certainly jump ahead to Chapter 3 (Habit 1) if you want. But I think that stopping here with me for just a few minutes will expand your understanding of *why* I'll be asking you to do certain things, and *how* you will gain momentum from each small change you decide to try to make. Knowledge is power, people. You need to know what goes on between your ears in order to control it!

When it comes to habit formation, there are two brain functions you need to understand. Not in detail, I promise. I'm obviously not a neurologist or a brain surgeon. This is just a 101 course.

YOUR GREEN BRAIN

The first Brain 101 lesson I want to impart concerns your body's fuel. Think of it this way: your body's gasoline is glucose. When you eat something, your body converts the carbohydrates in that food into glucose, better known as blood sugar.

The brain is a gasoline guzzler, the equivalent of a massive SUV. It consumes huge amounts of blood sugar; for its size it uses multiple times the amount used by other organs. But it's an SUV with a conscience. It tries to do its part to be green. It doesn't *want* to waste fuel.

Why? Well, your brain has a really long memory . . . all the way back to the hunter-gatherer days when humans couldn't go to the local gas station (supermarket) and fuel up with instant food. No, they had to hunt and gather and forage for every bite. So, as your brain sees it, food scarcity is a daily issue. It takes *great* pains to conserve energy. If it can

BRAINY VOCAB

Your brain is the most powerful muscle in your body. Forgetting for the moment that it is the organ that allows you to remember or forget something in the first place, never forget that your brain is the birthplace of all you do, say, and feel. I want you to swear to flex and care for your brain forever. Pay it some respect!

At this point there are only two brain regions you need to know. First, the medial temporal lobe. Scientists now believe that this chunk of the brain—located more or less in the center, at the bottom—contains many of the substructures needed for memory. These structures interpret signals from other organs—the eyes, the ears—and then coordinate with another brain component to make those memories into habits.

That other brain component is the basal ganglia, which sits close to the forebrain. It's positioned to receive signals from all around the brain. It then routes those signals to the right substructures.

use less blood sugar to help you navigate or deal with something, it will. As you'll understand better in a minute, the making of habits is a powerful way to conserve energy: instead of having to interpret anew an event or a smell or a sound every single time you encounter it, your brain draws on the memory of a past event, smell, or sound to direct an appropriate reaction.

HOW EXPERIENCES BECOME MEMORIES BECOME HABITS

If you were to look at brain tissue through a high-powered microscope while experiencing something—smelling a smell, hearing a sound, seeing the road in front of you—you would see neurons (brain cells) interacting. When two neurons experience the same sensory stimulation—that is, the event that's going on outside your noggin—they respond with a distinctly intense and unique chemical reaction. It's like a signature: the cells actually change to permanently internalize this new information, storing the memory-experience and reproducing it when signaled again by the same experience.

The brain also "chunks" memories, physically thickening the connection between the part where the experience is registered and the part where the memory is stored. The chunking process (yes, I swear that's a scientific term!) is like widening a freeway: everything moves along faster and easier. No traffic jams. No stopping and starting. Which every commuter knows saves fuel!

Author Charles Duhigg wrote a fascinating book called *The Power of Habit.* In it, he uses the terms *cue, behavior,* and *reward* to describe the stages of this neurological habit-making, fuel-saving process. Using his terms, consider the following scenario:

The first time you ever saw a stove, maybe you put your hand right there on that glowing red ring. This moment is "memorable" in the sense that you registered the pain of the heat, creating a unique chemical reaction between neurons and shooting some adrenaline into your system (you jump back and shout *ouch!*). The next time you experience the same thing, your brain remembers that first chemical reaction and draws on it again. This is a shortcut—and energy saver—for your brain: it doesn't have to waste fuel interpreting the experience for you anew each time; it can use the same chemical reaction and direct the same behavior.

And this is how you "learn" not to put your hand on a hot stove: the brain stores the memory of the pain you felt the first time, and triggers the warning the next time you're near a stove. You get the message "don't put your hand on the stove when it's red; be careful around hot things." That's your brain working in your best interest. And you're glad for that shortcut and that physical tingle of warning (the memory of that pain and adrenaline rush). Not putting your hand on a hot stove is a good habit to get into!

In the scenario above, seeing a red stove coil is the "cue" and it activates a behavior that has worked for you in the past (don't touch!), which leads to a reward (no burn, yay!). The behavior becomes habitual so long as the reward is meaningful to you (no burn = meaningful).

Let's look at the cue-habit-reward process in another situation: you see and hear a barking, slobbering, teeth-baring dog coming down the street at you. If the dog lunges at you or bites you or is memorably aggressive, that experience (the cue) is called upon the next time you encounter another dog: you remember that you should be on guard to avoid whatever happened last time (or to mimic the way you got away). Not being bitten is the reward.

Science has shown that a bad memory—a scary dog (or the burn from a hot stove)—triggers a certain kind of chemical reaction, one that is "stickier" than something that doesn't hurt or scare you. Really pleasant memories are "sticky" too—you tend to remember both happy and scary events from a long time ago better than an average day last week. But scary experiences—the kind that include pain or give you that adrenaline rush—stick the most. Yet again, there's an evolutionary reason for this that makes perfect sense: back in caveman days, humans needed to be vigilant about the dangerous and predatory things in their midst (woolly mammoths, saber-toothed tigers!). The brain therefore evolved to give preference to (and to chunk) lifesaving memories and warnings. So, now you understand that with the fang-baring dog memory, your brain is still doing you a favor.

But what if the second dog you come across is a sweetie like my dog Karl? If you let him, he'll give you a happy lick on your hand and an enthusiastic wag of his tail. There's nothing for you to be afraid of with Karl. But your brain sent you a different message when he first came into the room. You might have jumped back from him a little and started to sweat. Maybe you said, "Get that dog away from me!" Your brain was firing the same neurological reaction you had to the dog that tried to bite you last time. Together we might agree that you "overreacted," but no harm done (other than hurting Karl's feelings).

What happens the third time you meet a dog? You've now got these dueling memories—one dog tried to bite you, the other one was sweet. Well, remember that the frightening experience made more of a neurological impact, so you're probably going to remain wary. Maybe this time, before going anywhere near the third dog, you'll cautiously ask its owner if he's friendly.

Of course, if that third dog shreds the hell out of your fingertips you may be *scarred for life*! And what's "scarred for life" really saying? Your neurological association with dogs is now pretty set: you see a dog (the cue); your brain says it's appropriate to be nervous, maybe even to run the other way (the habit); and you avoid any new bites (the reward).

Even years later when you have had lots of pleasant experiences with dogs, that biter lingers in the back of your mind. Again, this is a smart neurological association, a prudent warning from your brain. Your experience tells you that it's a good habit to be cautious around dogs you don't know.

But this neurological memory-making process is *also* how you "learn" that a gallon of ice cream is the "appropriate" response to heartache or boredom or disappointment! Because when you eat and enjoy the ice cream (and its associated sugary rush of energy and pleasure), you *remember* that good feeling, which is the reward. Reach for ice cream a few times when "dealing with" disappointment and your brain is now "in the habit" of responding to that feeling with a self-soothing sugary treat. That neurological reaction is your brain's way of communicating, "You'll feel better if you pig out; get out a big spoon!" It's definitely not in your skinny interests to react to heartache or boredom with a gallon of ice cream every time.

All the more reason to be sure that you are conscious about the habits you are getting into. All the more reason to *redirect* the neurological paths your brain makes.

REROUTING THE CUE-BEHAVIOR-REWARD

How? Well, you need to make new habits. But before you speed ahead to find out what the most effective habits are—the six you'll start to read about in just a couple of pages—I want you to digest just two more key concepts.

First, understand that it is easier to *replace* a habit with a new one than to eliminate a habit altogether. Think about it—you need some kind of response to disappointment; you can't eliminate *having a response*. Cues are going to continue to pop up in your life, and you need a way to deal with them. *What your behavioral response will be* is the only piece of the cycle in your control.

Let's say you are in the habit of dealing with the stress of work parties by either hoovering up plates full of dessert or getting plastered. The cue is the stress of the social event, the behavior is to soothe your nerves with sugar or alcohol, and the reward is a combination of things: having something to do at the party besides dodge your boss, and the temporary sugar high (or buzz) that comes with the food and drink.

But this week you make a deal with yourself: whatever else you might do at the next party, you decide that you're going to talk to at least two new employees (who are probably more stressed than you, since they are new) *before* you go to the dessert table or the bar.

As you literally make yourself detour en route to the food and liquor—as you sidle up to the new guy from the mailroom to make polite conversation—the chemical signal of the new behavior detours energy that usually goes to the old head-to-the-food-and-booze routine. Your stop to chat makes the wiring of your old behavior wither just a bit. Energy gets diverted into storing the new experience and you're on your way to new wiring, and a new habit. Repeat the new behavior often enough and you chunk the wiring . . . and get a new habit cycle. Nicely done!

Second, the replacement behavior with the best chance of sticking and becoming a habit is one that gives you a really satisfying reward. I mean, you still need a moment on the other side of the cue that rewards whatever behavior or action you take.

Let's look again at the effort you're making to stop and talk to new employees before losing your cool at the office party. If that works for you, could it be that *talking to other people who are stressed* helps you feel less so? That is, could it be that the literal detour you make yourself take to talk to other nervous people calms *your* nerves? And once that's happened, you find you are less inclined to start doing shots and stuffing cake into your mouth? If so, you're on to something! Because the reward is actually the *calm feeling*.

Another example: let's say you want to replace your habit of stopping at Lou's Pizzeria on the way home from work on Fridays with the habit of getting some exercise instead. Other people tell you that the workout high you'll get is going to be reward enough for exercising. You suspect that's not going to cut it with you!

So now you need to really consider what it is about stopping at Lou's Pizzeria that feels good. Because you know deep in your heart that you actually feel a bit sick (physically) after all that cheese and dough and grease. And you know that you also feel kind of sick emotionally—disappointed in yourself every darn time you do it!

Think about this. Think about it hard. You know you are sort of celebrating the end of every long, hard work week by stopping at Lou's. And you like the welcome you get there—you've gotten to know the staff and they even know what your "regular" order is without your having to state it. Stopping at Lou's really isn't about the pizza, is it? It's a nice way to end every hard week—you find people who are happy to see you, and who ask no nagging or stressful questions.

Now that you are clearer on *why* you stop at Lou's Pizzeria, you can examine the options for replacing that behavior. You might find that going to the gym satisfies this need after a couple of weeks—you'll get to know the staff, and the instructor even congratulates you for showing up every time.

Nice people, no hard decisions (the instructor tells you *exactly* what to do!).

Or maybe you'll find that you really cannot stand to be shouted at in a boot camp or aerobics class every Friday night. You get that all week, thank you very much! But you still want exercise. So what about meeting up with a couple of friends to walk around the reservoir on Friday evenings? You can make plans for other kinds of end-of-week celebrations later in the evening, but you just might find that the walk (and friendly conversation) satisfies your end-of-the-workweek needs all by itself.

Long story short: you're probably going to have to tinker with things, try out new behaviors, and discover how rewarding they feel. But now that you know willpower is powered by belief, and you know the key interruption spot in the habit formation cycle, you *can* make these changes. You are ready to go!

three

HABIT 1:
MAKE CONTINGENCY PLANS

Have you heard the saying "The best-laid plans of mice and men often go awry"? How about "When we make plans, God laughs"? Both of these well-worn expressions are trotted out when we try and fail to control the circumstances of our lives. It's as though we're saying we just shouldn't bother trying to influence what is out of our hands. Fair enough . . . if you're talking about the weather or the economy or other people's behavior. You can't control those things and you'd be foolish to try.

But you'd also be foolish *not* to plan for how you will deal with even the most uncontrollable and unexpected things. There's a whole universe of things you *can and should* plan for, things that make your life easier and the world easier to navigate, especially when the going gets tough.

Like things you don't want to be surprised by: emergencies. Would you agree that it's wise to have batteries and candles in an easy-to-reach place in case you lose your power? And that it's prudent to have a jack and some flares in the trunk of your car so you're prepared if you get a flat tire? And it's smart to back up your hard drive, right? You can't control the storm or the nail on the road or the hacker who is intent on sabotaging lots of computers. But you can control your readiness for and reaction to these events.

Or you might plan for events that are a long way off, like your child's college education: even if you can't control where she'll get in, you can do a few things to improve her chances, like making sure she takes the SAT and gets some advice from her high school counselor on the kinds of schools to target. And though you can't know how much her college will cost or what portion of the tuition you'll have to cover (fingers crossed for that athletic scholarship!), you can and should *at least try* to save some money for the day when you do have to write a big old check.

You're with me so far, right? Making plans and thinking through contingencies *in advance* of their arrival is not futile. It's smart thinking.

So whywhywhywhy is it that when it comes to your health, you tend to drop the ball?

Does this describe you?

- You throw up your hands in defeat when you encounter a buffet table at a wedding or company party; you gorge yourself because "it all just looked so good" and you couldn't pull yourself away. Do you need a psychic to tell you there will be decadent food at those events? There's a time and place for being indulgent (see my Skinny Rule 20—you're allowed one splurge meal a week!), but every time you hit a buffet? Every single time? No! Believe it or not, there were plans you could have put in place that would have helped you go through the line only once.

- You don't get any exercise on vacation because, gee, you "forgot" your sneakers. Really? It was a surprise to you that there would be a gym at the hotel and/or that Florida in February would provide great walking weather? Again, there are times when you should cut yourself a break, and vacation might be the time to drop your regular workout routine and just relax. But that assumes that you have a regular workout routine.
- You regularly swear you're going to start to eat better and exercise more. Regularly, as in every New Year's Eve, right? How's that working out for you?

THE POWER OF CONTINGENCY PLANS

But of course, some people *do* have self-control and they *are* able to go through the buffet line only once (and pick the healthiest options), and they remember to bring sneakers and workout clothes when they travel (and use them while away!). On the outside—visible to you and me—they have *willpower.* And, no surprise, they are where they want to be, weightwise.

So what's the difference between you and them in the willpower department? What really explains a thin person's ability to keep temptation at bay?

As we discussed earlier, part of the difference lies in their *mindset,* their belief that they do have willpower in the first place. But in addition, it's the architecture of their *thinking*—which has been manipulated through their *contingency planning.* They have planned specifically and repeatedly and have made healthy decisions a habit; they've figured out the scenarios when they'll need an automatic response so they don't even need to think about what's best. That is, they don't have to *stop and think* or "exercise" self-control. It's become their default behavior.

Remember our lesson about the brain, fuel, and memory? Recall: the brain is stingy and would like to expend the least amount of energy possible. To save energy, your brain will always seek out the path of least resistance. And habits are the path of least resistance. They switch your behavior to default—for better or for worse—which conserves precious energy.

The operative phrase? *For better or for worse.* Obviously, there are good habits (habits that serve your higher goals of losing weight and getting in shape) and bad habits (habits that make you fat and unhealthy). If you are in the habit of going out to get a sugary snack in the late afternoon, your brain deals with your afternoon boredom (or your need to catch up on gossip with your sugary-snack-loving office-mates) by putting it in your head (literally!) that you should do what you always do: go on out and get that cake!

We humans aren't always rational (see Habit 3 for more on the irrationality of human decision making, especially at buffet tables!). We frequently make decisions that don't serve us well and take risks we shouldn't. But if you want to get or stay thin, you're going to have to override that irrational default behavior more often than not; you'll have to be more deliberate about planning in order to make good decisions easier for that tired old brain of yours.

But also remember, *you are not at the mercy of your current bad habits.* When you plan for challenges and situations—when you think about how you want to behave in situations that have always seemed to break your will in the past—you can create automatic new behaviors. You can plan in ways that will create new, good habits! Before you know it, choosing healthy, weight-loss-promoting behavior will become automatic, routine. This is what thin people do. They put their brains on weight-loss autopilot through contingency planning. Their consciously planned new routines override their bad ones.

YOUR BRAIN ON PLANS

Meet Peter Gollwitzer, a professor of psychology at New York University and probably the leading thinker when it comes to brain wiring and the psychology of motivation. He's done all the relevant studies on the complex attributes of habit formation and, more specifically, why most people make the wrong kind of plans. We have much to learn from him!

As a young psychologist, Gollwitzer became fascinated with the subject of goals, decisions, and intentions: How do we form them? Why do we act on them sometimes, and not others? Why do they seem so hard to alter?

For decades, psychologists who studied such things believed that the attainment of a goal was a reflection of just how badly one wanted the goal. But as Gollwitzer began experimenting, he soon saw that simply having a goal and really wanting to reach it *just ain't enough*. You know this all too well, right?

So he asked: What do people who *do* reach their goals do? What's their pattern? What do they do differently that makes them more successful than others?

Gollwitzer had a hunch: it was all about *clarity* and *detail* in one's goal plan. He saw that most people tend to focus on their big goal, without thinking through the subgoals and plans they'll need to get themselves there.

In one elegant experiment that tested his idea and proved his thinking, Gollwitzer and his fellow researchers recruited a group of college students who were getting ready to go on Christmas vacation. Before they departed for the usual sloth-a-thon of lounging at home, having mom make meals (and do laundry), and generally catching up on long-lost sleep, all of the students were assigned the task of writing a report on how they ended up spending Christmas Eve.

They were told to complete the report within forty-eight hours of Christmas Eve and send it back to Gollwitzer's team.

But . . . before they took off for vacation, half of the students were also asked to make a detailed plan for completing their report. They were instructed to write out *how, when, and where* they would complete their essay. In other words, they were asked to think about how they planned to implement their intention to complete the assignment.

The other half—the control group—were not asked to do the detailed planning.

The results were eye-opening: when the deadline arrived, three-fourths of the "implementation intention" students had written their reports; only one-third of the students in the control group had done so.

IF/THEN STATEMENTS

Gollwitzer and his team had pinpointed the helpfulness of "implementation intentions." That's kind of a mouthful, so I call this helpful planning strategy the creation of *if/then statements*. An if/then statement is basically a deal you make with yourself. As in: If I've got to go to the holiday party, then I'll hang out near the crudités; if I'm staying at a hotel, then I'll leave the key to the minibar at the front desk; if I've got a late morning meeting, then I'll tell the front desk to ring me early so I can go to the gym downstairs first.

You get the idea—you've got to think through and plan in ways that you know will help you reach your goal just as thoroughly as you would any other major endeavor in your life.

And the more specific and measurable, the better. Making vague, long-range plans like "I will drive across the country one day" is nice for daydreaming or creating a bucket list but is of dubious value when it comes to altering your day-to-day brain activity. As you saw above, all the science points to the effectiveness of shorter-term, specific plans.

Consider the office party you're heading to after work tomorrow. Which would you say is more specific and measurable? And which plan takes more brain energy to implement?

> **A:** "I will not overeat at the office party. I will not get drunk, either."
>
> **B:** "If there is a buffet at the office party, I will go to the cut-fruit platter first and fill up there at least three times before I eat anything else. I will also limit my alcohol intake to two glasses of white wine."

You know the answer! Plan B is certainly more measurable and specific. And though you might initially think the focus on counting drinks and plates of fruit takes *more* brain energy than the general admonition to behave, plan B is less work for your brain because it's a clear action plan. It gives you marching orders. No guessing. No brain straining.

The brain, ever the contingency expert, prefers already-mapped-out specific actions for specific situations, remem-

When you get specific about your plans—I will do X when confronted with Y—you allow the brain to conserve energy because you've decided your course of action ahead of time. When you do this repeatedly, you create a kind of neurological path that prompts automatic behavior, which conserves more energy. In other words, when you're in the habit of doing something, you don't *stop to think*, you don't hesitate. If you have worn a neurological path of instructions for what to order at your favorite Chinese restaurant, you don't have to read the whole menu. You are now in the habit of ordering your usual—chicken and vegetables, hold the rice, please!

ber? It can conserve energy through an *if X then Y* thought pattern. An overly vague, contingency-free plan requires you to constantly reassess (meaning many times over the course of the evening, in the office party scenario), and that is a serious drag on your brain energy. The lower your energy (the more mentally exhausted you become), the less reliable your healthy decision making.

Dr. Gollwitzer's research—in particular a recent meta review of ninety-four studies (some his own, many by others)—has found that the "if/then" habit-making process works with just about every kind of problem behavior in modern life, from smoking cessation to chronic lateness—even to recycling! Again, the more specific you can be in setting up if/then thinking, the better. It really works. Get ready to plan!

HARNESSING THE SUPERCOMPUTER
BETWEEN YOUR EARS

Now meet Heidi Grant Halvorson, a researcher at what I like to call the "laboratory of willpower," also known as the Motivation Science Center at Columbia University.

Like Gollwitzer, Halvorson and her colleagues have come to a similar and interesting finding: the brain basically operates in the way a supercomputer does as it sorts through the ones and zeros of a software program to make sense of it (and run it); your brain is an if/then contingency computer.

From the moment you were born, your brain has been taking in information, interpreting it, issuing an appropriate response based on past experiences (and past reactions to your behavior), and then filing the interaction away, saving the solution (your behavior) for use the next time a similar scenario presents itself. This is the essence of "learned behavior"—our kids learn from us what's expected and appropriate and file that away for future use. (Of course, as any parent who has ever sworn in front of a toddler knows, they can just as easily learn *in*appropriate behaviors— leading to an embarrassing situation when the toddler repeats mommy or daddy's colorful language in "similar" circumstances!)

As you grow and mature, you file away more and more if/then options, and you draw on them all the time. Over time, the brain gets better and better at "scanning" your environment for the *if*—a very specific cue—and faster and more efficient at implementing your new *then* routines.

And voila! Pretty soon, the if/then practice gives you a new habit—a powerful and unconscious connection between your own specific situation and your own specific response. Slowly but surely, as you apply your new *then*s to those old, familiar *if*s, you benefit from a kind of mental pause. As with any change—your new *then*s—there's a tiny halt of energy; this gives you an extra moment to inject your new tactic before you automatically shift to the old one. Call it an "Are you sure?" button. Let's use it!

THINK SMALL

Another way of thinking about being specific is to *think small*. I'm not talking about a smaller pant size (though I understand you want that too). No, I'm talking about breaking your BIG goal into smaller, more manageable—and measurable—ones.

Here's an example. On January 1 every year, thousands of people pledge to lose weight. Maybe that was you last year. You said: "I'm going to lose fifteen pounds by this time next year." That's a good goal. But if you didn't achieve it, it's probably due to the fact that beyond wanting to lose that weight, you didn't really make a plan to support that goal. You should have broken the goal down into subcomponents.

A little more detail might yield these statements to support the overarching goal: "I'm going to exercise more" and "I'm going to eat fewer carbs."

But of course, each of *those* intentions can be further bro-

ken down and addressed by another implementation intention. Consider exercise: one subgoal could be "I'm going to
take 10,000 steps a day," which could be further broken
down to "I'm going to buy a pedometer and take the stairs
at work."

You see what you're doing? You're creating a series of
smaller steps that will lead to the bigger goal. Then, for each
of these you'll write out an if/then plan.

Let's look at your weight-loss goal as a flowchart of goals
and subgoals:

I'M GOING TO LOSE 15 POUNDS BY THIS TIME NEXT YEAR.
(GOAL)
↓
To do that . . . I'm going on a low-carb diet.
(subgoal)
↓
To support that . . . I'll eat at least one vegetable at every meal.
(subgoal)
↓
To be prepared for that . . . I will buy at least one fresh vegetable over the
weekend and rinse, chop, and store it for use at meals throughout the week.
(subgoal)
↓
To make use of those veggies . . . I will try one new no-carb recipe a week.
(subgoal)

Now you've really got a plan to reach your goal!

THINK POSITIVE

How you phrase your if/then statement is important as well. And being positive is the key. When you use negative words (like *no, won't, don't,* or *shouldn't*), you are reinforcing/reminding yourself of the behavior you want to train yourself out of and forget. In other words, you want to emphasize the behavior you're going to *add* to your repertoire instead of repeating the behavior you need to stop.

That's why you want to say, "I'll take the stairs at work" instead of "I'll stop taking the elevator." Or, to use the example from the flowchart above, that's why you'll say, "I'll buy and chop vegetables" instead of "I'll stop eating so many carbs." This is a pretty simple adjustment—if you start being deliberate about it, it'll soon become second nature (a habit!).

CONTINGENCY PLANS IN ACTION

Scott Flanary is like a lot of young people who come to Los Angeles—or any big city. He came to get his career going in earnest, to discover new things and new friends. But big cities are also challenging places, and Scott wasn't the first to have adjustment issues and to have trouble coping with all the changes in his life. He started eating more than he should.

Scott had put on weight before, but now, forty pounds overweight, he fell into the fat-shame-regain cycle. As he

MAN'S BEST FRIEND
(and Woman's!)

Dr. Heidi Halvorson is not just some academic with a clip-board who studies motivation in a lab setting. She's got issues just like you and me.

As she tells it, "2003 was not a good year for me. It was the year that I turned thirty, separated from my first husband, and lived in near-constant dread of not finding a job before my postdoctoral funding ran out . . . I ate whatever I wanted, gave up completely on exercising, and rapidly packed on the pounds. I went out most nights to bars with friends and drank a bit too much. Some days I slept until noon. My apartment was a mess. My work suffered. I spent money impulsively, thinking new clothes and dinner at fancy restaurants would make me feel better, and blew right through my savings. It was the lowest point in my life, and I was miserable."

What turned things around? Something that required her to make contingency plans as though a life depended on her . . . because it did: she got a dog. The dog's very existence in her life demanded something from her: a new set of if/then plans to take care of him.

She had to make habits out of feeding and walking the little guy. She had to make time to play with him and groom him on occasion. And she had to be vigilant to keep him from chewing on her furniture and "prized possessions." As she says, "I was exercising a lot of self-control in order to care for this dog." And self-control in one area of a person's life—especially when you're feeling down or depressed about a lot of things—builds confidence, confidence that gives you the strength to take on other tough behavioral challenges. It's what you might call a "confidence cascade." You want that!

Think about Halvorson. She stumbled on a way to build healthier habits—even when she was surrounded by unhealthy stuff and temptation. Her if/then equations might have looked something like this:

"Even if I get home from work late, I will take the dog out for a walk."

"If the dog needs to chew on something, I will take him out to the park and find him a stick."

Soon, though, that way of thinking began to permeate her decision-making process in other problematic areas of her life. It didn't hurt, either, that she had a real-life, wriggling, barking bundle of fur reminding her to make him a priority! Using if/then implementations, she got her act together: her career took off again, she got healthy and lost weight, and basically she regained control of her life.

recalls, "I was single, unhappy, and fat. Something had to change."

At work, he experienced what so many of us experience: an unhealthy food environment, especially in terms of the local options for eating out. "Going out for a work lunch was impossible," he says. "It was always to a place with few healthy options—pizza, pizza, pizza!" And Scott likes pizza. Who doesn't? So, what were his options?

He might have planned this way: "*If* I go to that pizza place for a work lunch, *then* I will order a small pizza loaded with vegetables." Or "*If* I go to that pizza place for a work lunch, *then* I will drink two glasses of water to fill up before I take a bite of pizza."

But Scott was also trying to give up bread. And pizza dough is bread. He needed to formulate a plan not just to eat *less* pizza, but to eat something else entirely. He needed to get specific and he needed to phrase his intentions positively.

One day, looking over the schedule of office events—and contemplating how he'd get through them without putting on another fifty pounds—he got an idea. He decided what he needed to do was to stop being at the mercy of someone else's restaurant choice and change the venue when he could. He made a list of restaurants in the area that *were* healthy, that had menu items that would help him reach his goals. In if/then terms: "*If* it is suggested that we go to that pizza place for lunch, *then* I will refer to my list of healthier options and suggest one instead."

"I now have no trouble asking, you know, 'Hey where are we going? Can we try somewhere else?' It is a lot of front-loaded work, but it's worth it," he asserts. "Something is at stake. Eventually [being the guy to suggest a new spot] became part of my identity. Frankly, these days I have absolutely no problem being the guy who suggests something different and maybe a little less convenient. It's worth it."

Slowly but surely, Scott introduced his planning method to other challenges. "If I was going on a vacation, I researched the restaurants in the area," he explains. He even has a contingency plan for eating associated with dates: "If I'm going on a date, I'll actually pre-eat some dinner so I won't be so hungry when we order."

HABIT HOMEWORK

Get out a piece of paper and write down five or more of your own goals having to do with exercise and with food. Using simple arrows like I showed you earlier in the chart on page 34, break your goals down into as many subgoals as you can. Be specific and be positive.

Now that you are clear on your goals, it's time to imagine and think through the situations that might stand in your way. These are the scenarios for which you need to develop contingency plans. Drawing a blank? See the many ideas (collected from real people like you!) that follow.

Carry your food and exercise contingency plans with you (or on the note app on your phone) and add to them each time you find yourself in a new situation you hadn't imagined before. If it stands in the way of your reaching your goal, if it gives you trouble, you need a contingency plan for handling it.

If You're Drawing a Blank

Here are some positive and specific if/then statements to use if you want to eat better and exercise more. Do any of them give you an idea for your own life?

Contingency plans to help you meet your goal of eating better

> "If I get invited to a party where I know there will be snacks, I will allow myself to fill one small plate there, and that's it."
>
> "If I get a craving for something savory, I will eat a small handful of unsalted nuts."
>
> "If I go to the movies, I will bring chewing gum and chomp away as I walk straight past the popcorn counter."
>
> "If I am bored at home and looking for a snack, I'll do a yoga pose instead." (See pages 124–30.)
>
> "If I'm going food shopping, I will eat a healthy meal or snack before I go."
>
> "If I am fighting a food craving, I will drink a large glass of water immediately."
>
> "If I know I am going to be busy all day at work, I will pack small portions of nuts or an apple to eat in the event of salt/sugar cravings."
>
> "If I am invited out for a drink, I will order a white wine spritzer with lots of ice and drink it slowly."
>
> "If I know I am going to be busy all day, I will make sure I have a bottle of water next to me at all times."

"If I have a craving for a sweet drink in the evening, I will dress up a glass of fizzy water with sliced ginger, a squeeze of lime, or chopped fresh mint, or have a cup of hot tea."

"If I am at a birthday party and find myself holding a plate of cake, I will eat three small bites and put the rest in the trash."

"If I really must have chocolate, I will allow myself to eat four squares of organic dark chocolate that is at least 70 percent cacao."

"If I am at the store and considering buying something I shouldn't, I will read the ingredients label out loud from start to finish before I allow myself to buy it."

"If I feel sluggish after lunch, I'll *walk* to a coffee shop and get an espresso."

"If I am stressed and thinking about eating, I will close my eyes and take one slow, deep breath."

Contingency plans to help you meet your goal of exercising more consistently

"If I am driving to meet a friend for a meal, I will park a short distance from the restaurant so that I have to walk before and after the meal."

"If I am losing enthusiasm for my regular exercise class, I will take one new class a week at the gym for three consecutive weeks."

"If I am too tired to go to my regular exercise class, I will take a less strenuous one, like gentle yoga or a stretch class, instead of missing my workout altogether."

"If I'm ready for bed, I'll put my dog's chain and collar on the coffee table so I'm ready for a morning walk."

"If I am standing in line, I will stand on one leg for as long as I can and then switch sides."

"If I am sitting for long periods of time, I will set a timer and get up and take a short walk every hour."

"If I am going out for dinner with friends, I will tell them that I am taking up the Italian custom of going for a stroll after dinner, and invite them to join me."

"If I need to catch up with a friend I haven't seen in a while, I will find a fun exercise class to try and invite her to join me."

"If I feel sluggish, I will set a timer and try to hold plank pose for twenty seconds."

"If I need to have a long discussion with a friend, I will suggest we take a long walk together."

"If I need to come up with an idea for a date, I will suggest a hike or a walk along the beach."

four

HABIT 2:
CONSCIOUSLY PUSH BACK

I f you've done your Habit 1 homework, you now have some pretty strong if/then statements to help you work around and through goal-derailing situations. Good. Keep working that mental muscle and you *will* find yourself getting stronger and stronger in the face of temptations.

But let's be real. There will be times when you fall off the no-dessert or daily-exercise wagon. This is completely understandable. You know you're not going to have 100 percent compliance. Because you're not a robot, remember? Skinny people aren't perfect either!

What matters is how you deal with your inevitable slipups. Will you:

A: See your slipup as the latest sign that you are never going to be able to lose weight, that you are hopeless, that you might as well just give up now and have another brownie or milkshake or bowl of pasta or quit the gym, or will you . . .

B: Forgive yourself for your imperfections, tell your inner demons to go back to hell, and get on with the business of trying to toe the healthy-living line?

A is the automatic and irrational response. B is the considered and rational response. No surprise here: thin and healthy people choose option B. They understand that having two slices of that chocolate cake at last night's party was one and a half pieces too many, but it is *not the end of the world.* They are well aware that sitting on the couch all weekend bingeing on Netflix and popcorn did not live up to their fitness goals, but they *can get over it* and do better tomorrow (starting with developing a couple of new if/then strategies for party going or movie watching!).

So now, the obvious question: How can you wash yourself clean of your automatic/irrational responses and train yourself to be more considered and rational? Well, if shame is the feeling that sends you running back to old and comforting ways—to the refrigerator or the fast-food drive-thru or the living room couch—*conscious mental pushback* is the antidote. Pushback is the mental process through which you are going to shine a bright light on your irrational thoughts and analyze them for what they are and are not. And that, my friends, is something you can make a habit!

THE ROOT OF THE PROBLEM

First, though, let's step back and figure out what's going on when you're irrational. Maybe you're thinking: *The whole world is watching* or *Everyone thinks I'm such a loser.* What's irrational about either of those statements, of course, is that *the whole world* is not staring at you; that's physically impossible. And *everyone* really doesn't care so much about your personal life. Why do you let that kind of thought hijack reality?

Part of the answer is that you've likely created a neurological connection linking the experience of making a mistake to the reaction of shame; you've got a well-worn path in your brain for that kind of automatic thinking. And remember, once that groove is in place, your brain takes that shortcut to save energy.

Maybe you first started forming your personal brain path from slipup to shame way back when you were a child. Maybe an adult hollered at you and made you feel terrible about yourself once (or repeatedly). Or maybe there's someone in your life—a spouse, a boss, a "good" friend—who criticizes you all the time, and somewhere along the line you started to believe their hype.

There's no doubt that shame-filled, irrational thinking has root causes that might be found through formal psychotherapy (maybe years of it). And there's nothing wrong with trying to figure out the formative experience or access the memory at the root of it all. Knowledge is power! But while you're talking on the couch and wringing your hands and going through boxes of your shrink's tissues, you might also find it helpful to sit up and examine your thoughts from another perspective. Consider the wisdom of Dr. Aaron Beck—an Ivy League–educated clinical psychiatrist—who is considered the father of a psychological theory called cognitive behavioral therapy (CBT). I think of him as the Father of Pushback.

Early on, Beck seemed destined for a career in traditional psychotherapy, the kind where the patient lies on a couch and the psychoanalyst listens thoughtfully in a chair across the room, reflecting back and interpreting for the patient what he or she is hearing.

But one day, he had a profound insight. The patient on his couch had been telling him all about her sexual escapades and the anxiety she felt around them, and he'd been brilliantly psychoanalyzing the connection between forbidden thoughts and unconscious anxiety. They seemed to be making progress together. Above and beyond her happiness that they'd made some kind of breakthrough, she also seemed relieved.

"I was afraid that I was boring you," she explained.

Beck was surprised by this comment and seized on it. When he pressed her to tell him how long she'd been worrying that she was boring him, she admitted, "All the time." Furthermore, she revealed, "I think it when I am with you and when I am with other people." In other words, *worrying that she was a bore clouded this woman's every thought about herself!*

A lightbulb went off for him. As he later related the story: "It then occurred to me that there are two types of communication: internal and external. Internal refers to the automatic thoughts people have about themselves which they do not ordinarily share. On the other hand, thoughts usually communicated (i.e., external) in psychoanalysis are of the kind that people do communicate to other people." At this point, Beck realized that what we *don't say* out loud may be more useful than what we *do say*. He realized that our automatic thoughts propel us silently but powerfully. He realized he needed to help his patients get at those quiet, internal, automatic thoughts to help them change long-ingrained behavior. To do so, he explained, he would "sit them up [from the couch] so that we could talk back and forth." Cognitive behavioral therapy— the process through which doctor and patient find ways to *interrupt* those internal and automatic thoughts—was born!

It may seem so simple to us now, but what Beck was identifying was the vicious cycle of misinterpreted events leading to irrational thoughts. They are thoughts that provoke negative emotions and that lead to unhealthy behavior, which lead back to irrational thinking and so on. And even though Beck wasn't specifically concerned with weight loss, the cycle he pinpointed is, as you know, so so *so* problematic if you're trying to lose weight! The cycle looks like this:

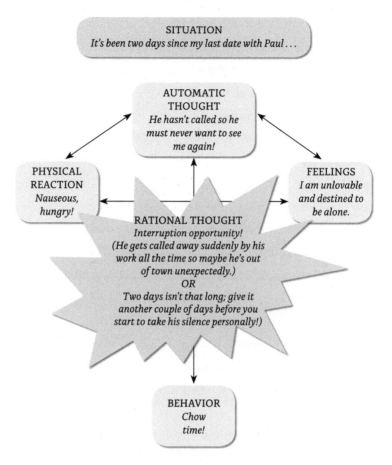

Feeling abandoned or unloved or insecure sends us rushing back to the harmful behavior that, in turn, sends us back into the shame cycle. Skinny people are able to interrupt the irrational connections between stressful or disappointing situations so that disappointment, regret, or even shame does not lead instantly to behaviors that will only make them feel worse.

UNDERSTANDING YOUR DISTORTED THINKING

As Beck looked for ways to put his insight into action with his patients, he returned to his basic proposition: regardless of where these automatic thoughts "originally came from" (traditional, long-term therapy's approach), their very presence in a person's life *now* was information enough to fundamentally tweak the way they interpret themselves and the world around them.

Eventually, he coined the term "cognitive distortion" to describe the way our automated thoughts can quickly turn irrational. And over time, he came up with a list of common forms of cognitive distortion, many of which overlap and feed into others.

Again, knowledge is power. Getting to know these fifteen common thought processes is the first step toward interrupting them. Check out the list below—these aren't the technical psychological terms that Beck used, but the gist of the types are intact. See yourself in any of the examples?

1. Using a Bad Filter

You see all the negative details, totally blow them out of proportion, and don't even bother considering the positive aspects of a situation.

Example: Susan has been working hard at her exercise program for six months. She checks her progress on the scale and in the mirror every morning. She is definitely losing some weight and her arms and legs are looking more

YOUR BRAIN ON SHAME

In 2010, researchers at England's Aston University made a discovery that shines a little more light on what's going on in that head of yours when you experience shame. The researchers took scans of the brains of people they'd exposed to critical, denigrating self-talk. In essence, they were shaming these people and then seeing the effect on brain activity. The imaging hot spots (showing the parts of the brain being engaged) appeared in the regions known as the left lateral orbitofrontal cortex, the left lateral prefrontal cortex, the dorsolateral prefrontal cortex, and the inferior temporal cortex. You can look up those fancy scientific terms if you like. Or you can take my word for it that these regions have been linked to what are called "error processing" and "defensive states"—either anxiety (fight) or depression (flight). Simply put, to the brain, coping with the emotion of shame is similar to being anxious or depressed. Talk about thinking unhappy thoughts!

By contrast, when the same researchers exposed their subjects to self-reassuring, complimentary self-talk, distinctly different parts of the brain lit up. This time, the imaging hot spots appeared in the left temporal pole and the insula, regions usually linked to empathy and compassion for others. The brain uses the same areas when exercising self-compassion as it does when being compassionate or kind to others.

Knowing this, and knowing that you can actually manipulate your brain by being deliberate about the quality of your self-talk, why would you ever talk to yourself so unkindly? What would you say to your best friend if she confided in you that she'd just binged on unhealthy food for a whole weekend? Wouldn't you tell her to forgive herself and get back to healthier living without a glance back at the caloric, slothful weekend? Yes, you would.

Okay, would you cut yourself the same kind of slack? Probably not. But you will learn to. What you think about yourself is true, so think kind thoughts.

toned than ever, but her midsection isn't as slim as she would like it to be. Instead of acknowledging her progress (which would make her feel good about herself and give her more energy), she focuses on the size of her waist, letting that "problem spot" be the filter for interpreting the success (or failure) of her efforts. This makes her feel depressed and she starts losing enthusiasm for her workout.

2. Black and White Thinking

You can't see the gray areas of a situation. You're either perfect or you're a failure. No middle ground!

Example: Jane has followed her diet successfully for three weeks, but she slips up and has one cookie during an office meeting. Instead of seeing that cookie as an isolated bump on an otherwise very smooth road (three weeks of diet adherence!), she takes an all-or-nothing view of her failure; she allows that one cookie to derail her completely. All is lost! She eats another five cookies at the meeting, and picks up a pizza and a tub of ice cream on the way home for dinner.

3. Overgeneralizing

If something bad happens once, you think it will always be that way.

Example: Steve has been diligent with his diet and exercise program for a while. He has lost weight and he is looking good, but he still worries that he is not attractive to women. He summons up the courage to ask a woman out on a date. It is a pleasant evening, but it is obvious that there is no sexual chemistry between them. Instead of acknowledging that this is perfectly natural (sexual chemistry can't be sparked with everyone) and gaining confidence from being back on the dating circuit, he jumps to the conclusion that women are simply not attracted to him. He tells himself that he will *never* find love because he is too fat and too ugly. Shame sets in. He doesn't go on another date for a year.

4. Mind Reading

You think you can divine what people think about you and why they act the way they do. And without any evidence!

Example: Lindsey is shopping for a new outfit to inspire her to stay on track with her diet. She finds a pair of jeans she loves, but she can't find her size. She approaches a saleswoman and asks if they have her size in the back. A minute later, she sees the saleswoman talking in hushed tones to another person who works in the store. They are both glancing over at Lindsey. The two saleswoman are actually discussing whether they can give Lindsey the pair in her size they know is on hold in the back (a pair stashed there for one of the saleswomen's sisters), but Lindsey assumes that they are talking about her weight and laughing at her size. She leaves the shop in shame before the saleswoman can return with the good news that they do have one pair left!

5. Inflating/Catastrophizing

You totally blow everything out of proportion. You expect the worst out of any given situation.

Example: John has been on a new exercise regimen for three months. He is starting to feel great, and he is enjoying the new muscle definition in his arms and shoulders. One day, he bench-presses a little too enthusiastically and feels a slight twinge in his shoulder. The next day his shoulder is a bit sore so he decides to take a couple of days off. Then he starts obsessing. He keeps moving his arm to check if the pain is still there, which in turn aggravates the sore spot. He researches shoulder anatomy online and starts panicking that he has a rotator cuff injury that will immobilize him for months and turn him back into a weak-armed fatty. Feeling totally disillusioned, John stops going to the gym altogether.

6. Judge and Jury

You think that everything people do or say is some kind of reaction (usually bad) to you. Then you compare yourself to others and set up an idea against which to unrealistically judge yourself.

Example: Anne is looking for somebody to help her keep up her fitness goal of walking for one hour twice a week. Anne invites her coworker, Lucy, to join her for a walk. During the walk, Lucy tells Anne that she regularly runs marathons. Anne is mortified; she assumes that she is slowing Lucy down and is convinced that Lucy is bored. When Lucy tells Anne how much she is enjoying walking and chatting, Anne doesn't believe her. Anne spends the rest of the walk worrying that Lucy thinks she is fat and unfit and comparing her legs unfavorably to Lucy's.

7. Control-ism

You must be in control, even over things that you really can't reliably control! If you can't, you feel that you have failed, that you are weak, and you lapse into a shame-binge cycle.

Example: Ken is struggling to keep to his gym routine. One recent morning all he really wanted to do was lie down in the garden and read, but he made himself get into his workout gear and drive to the gym. On the way, however, his car broke down. Rather than get mad at the manufacturer or his local mechanic, Ken got burning mad at *himself.*

Convinced that it was all his fault—that he "must have" been irresponsible in maintaining the car (even though he's very responsible about it)—he shouted at the sky, "Typical me!" He finally phoned for roadside assistance, but since his routine was out of whack, he walked to a nearby donut shop while waiting for help to arrive. One donut became two . . . and so began the binge.

8. The Fairness Delusion

You feel you know what is fair in most situations. If others disagree or behave in what you would consider "unfair" ways, you are resentful. You feel resentful because you think you know what is fair but others won't agree with you.

Example: Tina goes over to her friend's house for lunch. She brings a veggie salad and a big bunch of grapes. Two other friends who are healthy and thin are also invited. One of them brings a big bag of potato chips and the other brings a box of cupcakes. They tuck in enthusiastically, exclaiming how much they enjoy "naughty" treats and a good gossip. Tina resents this, as they know she is on a diet. Tina claims that it is not fair that she should have to watch them eat the goodies while she deprives herself, so she joins in.

9. Blame-Gaming

Someone is always to blame. You hold other people responsible for your pain, which is—let's face it—not always rational, or, worse, you blame yourself for everything.

Example: Ellen is a single mother of two young children and she has been struggling with her weight for a long time. Her doctor told her that if she doesn't start exercising, she is likely to suffer health complications. She wants to be the healthiest mother she can be for her children, so she resolves to go to the gym on Monday morning and sign up for some sessions with a personal trainer. On Monday morning, one of her children is sick, so she has to drop him at her mother-in-law's house. There is a terrible accident on the freeway, and she gets stuck in traffic for an hour. She misses her time slot at the gym and has to go to work instead. She blames herself for failing to start her exercise program and feels like a bad mother.

10. The "Should" Illusion

You have a secret list of many inflexible commandments and rules about how you and others should act. You blame yourself if you break the rules, and others if they do—even if they have no clue about your "shoulds."

Example: Dave was in a car accident ten years ago that has left him with ongoing back pain. He also has high blood pressure from excessive alcohol consumption, and he pushes himself too hard at work. Dave wants to start exercising and his doctor recommends that he take up yoga to help with his back issues and reduce his stress levels. Instead of finding a gentle class that is appropriate for his age and his health issues, Dave takes a power yoga class because his internal "commandments" stipulate that he *should always* be able to take on the toughest of challenges. Dave forces himself into difficult positions that are way beyond his ability and does something to his back. As he hobbles out of the studio he thinks: *I should have been able to do that easily. What's wrong with me?* Feeling more stressed than when he went in, he swears off more yoga.

11. Making Feelings into "Fact"

"What I feel must be true." If you feel fat, you are. If you feel stupid, you are.

Example: Jill recently discovered that she has a sensitivity to dairy; milk and yogurt and ice cream and cheese all make her feel really bloated and gassy. Since she's been avoiding dairy products, she's lost quite a lot of weight and looks and feels fabulous. For her birthday, she and her husband go out to a little Italian restaurant they've been wanting to try. They have a great time, laughing away and planning a vacation for the following year to Italy. Caught up in the festive mood, she decides to "treat" herself to a pizza with fresh mozzarella and also a gelato for dessert. On the drive home, Jill starts to feel bloated and lousy. She loosens her belt. Forgetting that the cheese and gelato might have been the source of her problem, she registers that she is getting fat. Her spirits plummet, she gets into an argument with her husband, and the next day she goes off her no-dairy plan again . . . and again and again.

12. *The Change Delusion*

You think other people will always change just because you pressure or "convince" them to do so. If they don't change, your hopes for happiness are dashed.

Example: Pam and Geoff are retired and they do everything together. They visit their grandchildren, go to movies, grocery shop as a team, and even read the same books so they can talk about them together. One of their favorite things to do is go out for indulgent lunches. Needless to say, they are both on the heavy side. Pam is more bothered by this than Geoff, and she suggests that they change their eating patterns and introduce daily walks into their routine. Geoff vehemently resists, telling Pam that he wants to carry on enjoying life as they have been doing. "Life's short!" he exclaims. "We should be doing what we want at our age!" Pam makes the argument that their lives will be longer and happier if they are healthier. But Geoff refuses to change. Instead of making her own changes within their routine— such as ordering salad at lunch instead of pasta, and going off for a stroll in the afternoons while Geoff is napping— Pam concludes that it is useless to try without Geoff, and she gives up on the idea of being healthy.

13. *Global Labeling*

You generalize one or two qualities into a negative judgment that must apply to everyone all the time.

Example: Deborah grew up in a military family and was

raised by strict parents. Deborah's sister, Tessa, flourished and became a sergeant major in a Marine Expeditionary Unit. Deborah, meanwhile, struggled with her weight and showed an incredible flair for decorating cakes—an ability whose value was lost on her parents. Eventually Deborah moved away from home to pursue her dream of opening up a cake shop. As part of her new life, she decided to join a local weight-loss support group. She was hoping to be inspired, but as she sits looking at the overweight people in the room, she finds herself judging them for being weak and lacking in willpower. She concludes that support groups are all "just for losers." She leaves the meeting, trying to convince herself that she should be able to lose weight by herself.

14. Perfectionism

You see everything through the lens of being right all the time. You put yourself on trial to prove that your opinions and actions are correct.

Example: Tom is an overachieving lawyer and a junk food addict. When he starts dating a girl at work, he decides it is time to start eating healthily and taking care of his appearance. He researches all of the latest diets and exercise programs and devises for himself an austere regime of juice fasting and long-distance running. When Tom's girlfriend questions the extremity of his choices and complains that he doesn't spend enough time with her because he is always out running, Tom insists that he has come up with the perfect way to achieve optimal fitness. She tries to point out that his regime is not sustainable, but he won't listen and he accuses her of trying to undermine his efforts. She breaks up with him. Tom brands himself unlovable and relapses into eating junk food.

15. The Atta-Boy "Rule"

You expect that all of your sacrifices and hard work will be constantly rewarded with praise (either verbal or some kind of tangible award). If you don't get that praise or accolade, you both resent others and denigrate yourself for "failing."

Example: Jenny holds herself to a very high standard in all areas of her life. She has a well-paying job, a great husband, and a beautifully kept house. She works out religiously and prides herself on looking good. She often gets compliments from complete strangers. Jenny and her husband decide to have a child and, at age forty-two, she gives birth to twins. She returns to her workout routine as soon as she can and continues to eat healthfully. But, try as she might, she cannot shift the last layer of "baby fat" and is dismayed to look in the mirror and see bags around her eyes. She is not turning heads like she used to and concludes she is unattractive. She resents her best friend, who is younger and who bounced back very quickly after giving birth. Jenny punishes herself for being a failure and begins to distance herself from her husband. She starts skipping her workouts and turning to food for comfort.

INTERRUPTING YOUR DISTORTED THINKING

Tired of reading all those irrational thoughts and thought distortions? Recognize yourself all too many times? Ready to start interrupting that nonsense and push back? Yes, yes, yes, Bob!

Okay, it's time for you to do a little research. Before you get all hot and bothered and toss this book aside because you're sensing *work,* let me assure you that I'm not talking about the kind required to write a term paper.

The kind of research I'm talking about is the collection of information (facts, evidence, actual past experiences) that overrides the old, subjective messages you've created and repeated to yourself. In other words, you're just going to step back a little from the situation, observe the illogic of your thoughts, and interject a rational thought or two that will interrupt the negative self-talk just long enough to put your thoughts on a slightly different path. A positive path. A self-compassionate path. A path that will soon wear a new and positive and healthy and self-compassionate groove into your brain! Voila—there's your Skinny Habit.

Here is a classic example of the slip-shame cycle and the three steps you need to take to stop it in its tracks:

Situation: You have just weighed yourself and, unfortunately, you've put on two pounds.

Now, inevitably and understandably, you are going to feel a variety of things: shame, frustration, fear of rejection, impotence, weakness, anger about the unfairness of it all. And then you're going to have your own brand of negative automatic thoughts. Maybe: "Everyone will notice at the beach party tomorrow and be talking about it at the office on Monday." Or maybe, "Oh crap! No matter what I do, I fail."

STEP 1: Note the automatic thoughts you have immediately after the situation: "Great. Another example of my weakness!"

STEP 2: Pause and just note what emotions you feel. This doesn't take more than a second. Just make a mental note! The simple act of observing your own thought pattern is sometimes enough to shift things right away.

STEP 3: Looking over the preceding list of fifteen common thought distortions, try to pinpoint which one (or ones) are in evidence here. What's the unconstructive mental pattern at play? Here again, just labeling the insanity can be enough to snuff it out. But let's make sure, okay? Move to step 4.

STEP 4: Interject at least one fact that counters the distortion. For example: "I've put on two pounds before and I have lost it again pretty fast." Or, here's a "fact-based" statement that's perhaps not quantifiable in a lab but is based on what we all know to be true: "Everyone is a little self-conscious in a bathing suit, which means that everyone will probably be focused on themselves and not me." Or use the "catchall" pushback: imagine what you'd say to a friend in the same situation. Would you tell her she should be ashamed of herself, or would you encourage her not to see this as more than what it is: a temporary setback?

The game changer in this process is the rational and self-compassionate information you use as ammunition. In the Habit Homework, you're going to be proactive about stockpiling that ammunition! I think you'll be amazed at how quickly this averts the slip-shame-binge cycle. You'll feel calmer and more in control already. The renewed self-reassurance will start lighting up the brain regions you *want* to engage instead of those competing self-critical regions!

Thought Interruption in Action

When I first met her on the set of season eight of *The Biggest Loser,* Amanda Arlauskas was an energetic and determined nineteen-year-old from New Jersey. Amanda eventually placed third on the show, losing 87 pounds, going from 250 pounds to 163! She was a truly inspirational young woman.

After she left the show, however, Amanda went back to the same world she'd gotten overweight in. Since it was New Jersey—pizza central—there was saucy, cheesy temptation around every corner. Furthermore, she felt like she was "living in a snow globe" and that people who recognized her from the show were scrutinizing her every move. "Anywhere I went, people were sizing me up. You know, like *What is she wearing?* and *What is she eating?* and *Is she getting fat?*"

With the stress and the opportunity to binge on a food she loved, Amanda regained forty pounds.

Let's break this down so far: She *had a slip*—the stress eating of pizza. She started to really beat herself up mentally. Those thoughts and feelings aroused and reinforced destructive beliefs she had about herself. So she ate more. She gained more. As she put it: "I had a total meltdown. I was thinking, *What is wrong with me? Will I always be screwing up?* All of my demons came back." All along, her thoughts were distorted: she was guilty of mind reading (*Everyone thinks I am getting fat*) and telling the future (*I will always screw up*), and she was also blinded by the "should" illusion because she felt *The Biggest Loser* had given her the tools to deal better with temptation and weight gain.

But then one day, Amanda had a revelation that routed her thoughts in another direction. She saw a photo of herself taken when she was lighter. She noted that she looked pretty damn good in that picture, and she liked that look. She *remembered* being that size. "I started thinking, you know, *that's* me! That's the person I really am." And when she put on her "skinny clothes," she could see that she could still fit into them, if not totally comfortably. She started to realize that she was still within striking distance of her weight goals. All was not lost!

As she describes it: "I realized I had been thinking, *I'll never get slim again. I'm so weak. I'll always be alone.* But in reality I had 'skinny clothes' that kind of still fit and I had a boyfriend who thought I still looked great." She used those rational views of herself to override the older, irrational thinking. When she was feeling down about the slow climb back to her *Biggest Loser* best, she recalled the facts: she'd managed to keep weight off for long periods of time before; her clothes still fit; she had photos to prove she'd met her goals in the past; by all signs her friends loved her. "I felt better, ready to tackle all the demons that always go off in my head!"

What about all those people sniping at her? Amanda got rational about that as well: "Let's face it—most people are just too self-centered to even notice others, let alone form a reasonable judgment."

Eventually Amanda lost the weight and kept it off. It was not easy. "I realized then that I had to force myself to do something when the demons came back. I had to tell myself, 'No, that is *not* me! The facts say something different, Amanda. *You made a mistake, but you're not a failure.*'"

HABIT HOMEWORK

Now that you understand the process of pushing back, you probably need to practice this conscious interruption process. You'll definitely need to arm yourself with some rational ammunition you can fire at your destructive thoughts!

STEP 1: To get started, think of a recent real event and/ or typical situation that would send you spiraling downward. Imagine the situation: What, exactly, with no embellishment, happened?

BONUS HOMEWORK

Keep a running list of rational pushbacks on your computer or on the note-taking app on your phone. Better yet, print out or write out some of your best one-liners and put them where you'll see them when you need them—on your bathroom mirror, on the refrigerator door, on your workout clothes drawer, on the kitchen door! These rational reminders of your own power and of your own positive experiences will slow you down from breaking your if/then promises to yourself!

STEP 2: Now write what you automatically *thought*. Got that noted? Great.

STEP 3: How did that automatic thought make you *feel*—physically and emotionally? Make a note, mental or otherwise.

STEP 4: Look at the list of common thought distortions on pages 49 to 60. Pick out the ones that seem to underlie your negative automatic thoughts. You get it. It's like inventorying your main mistakes and giving them a name. You'll start to see a pattern. Believe me, you'll start to see a pattern.

STEP 5: Now for each irrational thought/thought distortion, try to imagine what you'll say to yourself the *next time* such a situation occurs.

five

HABIT 3: REENGINEER YOUR ENVIRONMENT

I n *Skinny Rules* I offered lots of simple strategies for implementing some of my twenty "nonnegotiable principles for getting to thin": putting a glass of water by your bedside so it's the first thing you drink when you throw your legs over the side of the bed each morning, or placing the healthiest snacks at the front of your refrigerator or at eye level in your cabinets so they're the easiest things to reach for when you go snack hunting. These are small but really meaningful ways to make common behaviors (getting up in the morning, eating whatever you see first) work in your skinny favor. They are ideas for *reengineering* your immediate surroundings in ways that support your efforts to stay on the rules. (They can also be phrased as if/then contingency plans to support your goals to follow the rules.)

But the idea of reengineering your *environment* to get or

stay healthy and trim needs to go beyond simple tricks to set yourself up for success. Actually, the idea of environment is what we need to expand on here.

Am I talking about clean air? Ozone protection? Global warming? All important civic concerns, and all obviously have an impact on the health of the planet, the atmosphere, your hemisphere, and the little patch of local land you call home. And ultimately, of course, a healthy environment in the global sense has a positive impact on your physical health as well. But while I'm sure there are a lot of thin environmentalists out there, being "green" isn't what I'm referring to here. (Just saying: there are a lot of not-so-thin environmentalists, too.)

In the context of the behavior that thin people have made a habit, I use the word "environment" to refer to two important aspects of your world: your *social environment* and your *built environment.* Think of these two environments as the scaffolding in your life; the architecture of your day, they comprise the people you see and interact with and the things you see, say, and do. And remember, the things you see, say, and do repeatedly have a significant impact on the architecture of your brain: they create neural pathways that make your thoughts and behavior into habits. So you see where I'm going with this, right? If you were paying attention to the chapter heading, you've made this leap in logic already: thin people manipulate their environment to create patterned behavior (aka habits) that supports their weight goals and/or their achieved thinness. They reengineer their surroundings to reinforce healthy habits.

Your *social environment* is made up of the people you hang out with and the things you do together socially. Your *built environment* is composed of the physical things around you, both macro and micro in nature—from the color of your room to the number of fast-food restaurants near your work to the placement of your refrigerator or snack drawer at home.

YOUR SOCIAL ENVIRONMENT

Whom do you live with? Who are your closest friends? What about the people you work with—what are they like? These people, and the things you all do together, are the substance of your social environment. These people influence you (with and without your knowledge) and impact your weight and your ability to control your weight more than you might have ever considered.

Try this little assessment about how healthy your social environment really is: What do you and your friends or family do together with your common downtime?

Do you . . .

Exercise?
Go clubbing?
Cook?
Sit quietly and read books?
Binge-watch television shows while eating ice cream?
Drink heavily?

Bottom line: Do you consider that you're good influences or bad influences on each other?

I know what you're thinking: no one has friends and family members who are *always* one or the other, always a good or bad influence. Instead, you probably have people in your life who are a little of both. The same person who claims to support your attempts to lose weight and is willing to do things that will make both of you healthy is sometimes more than happy to drive you to the convenience store for more chocolate chip cookie dough ice cream at 11 P.M. and/or order another round of shots (without paying!). No one is *always* either an angel or devil on your shoulder.

But for purposes of adopting healthy Skinny Habits, you need to start looking at your relationships a little more critically. When you do, you'll start to see patterns of collective behavior: Your wild clubbing/drinking nights are most often with your buddies Eric and Tom. You and Sheri tend to bring out the pig-out-and-binge-watch-TV thing in each other. Funny, but now that you think of it, it's Michael and Joanne you tend to pair with to walk the dog. And when it's Jen coming over for dinner, you find yourself trying a new recipe from *Skinny Meals* instead of making your grandma's fettuccine Alfredo with cream and loads of cheese and breadsticks (Eric and Tom get *that* meal).

The Science of Social Environments

Still don't completely believe that your buddies impact your health and still need convincing to reengineer your social surroundings? Consider this: believe it or not, scientific evidence is now mounting that obesity can be transmitted, kind of like a contagious disease! Yes, spending time with heavy people can make you heavier yourself.

If this were a movie, you would have just done a double take and the soundtrack would have been the squealing brakes of a car, right? But it's true. Read on.

In 2007, a group of Harvard researchers became very interested in how social networks—from family to coworkers to good friends—factor into the obesity epidemic we were then (and still are) experiencing in this country. Reviewing data collected for the famed Framingham Heart Study—three decades' worth of health information kept on a huge group of people who had volunteered to be studied for heart health research—the researchers started to see patterns and correlations that they had not originally been looking for. The Framingham data not only collected health information every year on the people being studied but also incidentally asked each person to report on the general health (including weight) of their siblings and spouses over time as well.

What they found was remarkable: a person's chances of becoming obese increased by 57 percent if he or she had a friend who had become obese. If a person's sister or brother was or became obese, the person was 40 percent more likely to become obese as well. For spouses, the number was a tiny bit lower, but still significant: 37 percent.

Of course, there's no blood test or MRI that can tell us exactly why this phenomenon occurred, but one explanation was offered: we take on the behaviors and/or the mind-set of the people we spend time with.

Forgetting the off-the-charts-wacky couple of friends that each of us has (you know you do!), you probably think your friends are pretty normal, right? And not counting crazy Uncle Joe and your family's particular nuttiness, you likely think your family is the norm as well, yes? The logic goes that if those friends or family members are obese, and you are around them a lot, you are likely to consider being fat not only as acceptable, but as normal since it's all around you.

Even if we don't think their weight is "normal" and we don't want to look like them, we often unwittingly take on the behaviors that made that friend or family member obese in the first place: overeating together or being too sedentary when you hang out. Either way, it seems that our friends and family are our visual and behavioral *cues*. Or, as the Harvard researchers concluded: "People are connected, and so their health is connected."

Does this mean you are doomed to be or stay fat if your social network is fat? No, but it does mean making some changes. It means that you need to *also* have strong emotional bonds with people who have Skinny Habits. You must make more consistent relationships with healthy people doing healthy things to offset the less-than-healthy influences of others.

If you want to get or stay at a healthy, happy weight—the weight that makes you proud to strut your stuff and the weight that makes you comfortable in your own skin—you're going to have to get your head around this: the people you surround yourself with have an amazing impact on your weight and weight control.

How to Reengineer Your Social Environment

Meet Danny Cahill. I first met Danny on the set of season eight of *The Biggest Loser*. He was 430 pounds then and, understandably, pretty depressed about his weight and his health. As he recounted later, "I remember feeling hopeless, like a person with a $100,000 debt and a $40,000-a-year job."

Danny ended up winning that year, getting himself down to about 191 pounds (a loss of 239 pounds!).

And Danny kept most of that weight off for about a year by continuing the good eating and exercise habits he'd learned on the show. A year or so after returning home, however, the going got tough. There were the endless responsibilities of his business, his family, and his service commitments. It wasn't that he was surrounded by people who were necessarily bad influences on his desire to keep his weight off, but he was surrounded by an atmosphere that hampered his ability to do and choose healthy things.

As he put it: "I struggled with the stress environment."

As I put it: his social environment was weighing him way down (and rocketing his weight way up).

But then things went from tough to worse: his father died, and he was devastated. In the weeks and months that followed his father's passing, he let go of any remaining healthy eating and exercise routines. He went back up to 290 pounds and "was back to filling my soul with food. I realized I had to do something."

Danny understood that exercise is both a good way to burn calories and a great stress buster, so he knew he could kill two birds with one stone if he could find a way to get back into an exercise routine. He knew from his experience on *The Biggest Loser* that seeing some positive results on the scale through exercise would spur him to eat better and better, too. He later did a few things in his physical/built environment to cue healthy living (more on those strategies shortly), but at the time and with all he had on his plate, he just couldn't seem to get an exercise routine going again on his own. At his lowest point he realized, "I had to reach out. I realized I couldn't do it myself."

He had to reach out. That's such a telling statement to me. He needed to get back to the atmosphere of teamwork and camaraderie he felt while on *The Biggest Loser.* While there he'd been with other people trying to reach similar goals and he'd been supported in reaching his own; he had been on a team and was spurred on daily by the sense of being in the competition together.

So, what did Danny do to reengineer his social environment? "I re-created some of that sense of urgency I'd had on

> Reengineering a healthy social environment boils down to this: you must make more consistent relationships and bonds with healthy people doing healthy things.

the set. We didn't have a lot of money, so I made myself a deal. I took out a six-month membership at a gym. I'd be wasting it if I didn't use it." That's what did it—he joined a gym to be around others who wanted to be healthy. He joined a gym even though the expense was a pinch on his budget. He actually used that budget discomfort to spur his attendance. Kind of brilliant. And so simple.

Joining healthy people doing healthy things also helped my friend Mark Kruger. Mark has lost 120 pounds—he looks amazing! But one of the things he discovered quickly was that he needed to "take away the excuses" that might lead to regain. There was one classic thought pattern/excuse that could cause him problems: the old *everyone else is doing it, so why shouldn't I?* logic. Or, as he put it: "All my friends do it; how do you expect me to resist?"

Looking at this from a reengineering perspective, I hope you see what I see: Mark had put his finger on what was going to trip him up (spending time with people who didn't want or didn't have to resist unskinny habits) and that led him to one uncomfortable conclusion: "I couldn't go back to the same people who enabled my bad habits."

But having the epiphany didn't necessarily mean Mark had to cut those friends out of his life. They may have been bad influences in some respects, but they were still his friends! Instead, Mark shifted his schedule a bit and spent more time with a group of friends who espoused better weight and fitness ideals.

"I got into a workout group that met in the morning. You've got to show up if people are there waiting for you. It's not fair for you to sleep in while they're waiting. So I get up. I know they're there. Being around like-minded people and keeping the routine: that's the key."

Or, like the Harvard guys said: "People are connected, and so their health is connected."

Relax: reengineering your social environment doesn't require divorcing your spouse or de-friending your drinking buddies! Sometimes the best fix is to *add* friends (not take them away) or just have a change of scene. Look at the Habit Homework on page 84 for ideas that will help you assess your roadblocks and temptations and then reengineer your personal solution!

YOUR BUILT ENVIRONMENT

Take a minute to think about how often you have to make a decision about food on a given day. It's not just at breakfast, lunch, and dinner, but all the hours in between: what to put in your shopping cart for this week's meals; tall, grande, or venti at the coffee shop; what time to meet your mom for brunch, where to sit when you get there, and what you'll order off the menu. But that's just the obvious stuff! Would you believe that on average, you make 250 food-related decisions every day? It's true! Though you might not be aware of it, you never really stop having to think about what to put in your mouth and how you'll do it (volume, speed, heat, spice . . . so many decisions!).

Unfortunately, your physical surroundings—both the big, structural things (macro surroundings) and the small details (micro surroundings)—undercut Skinny Habits and healthy decisions in very subtle ways all the time. Part of the reason for this is that your built environment is often built by people and companies that want to sway you one way or another! Supermarket managers, food manufacturers, restaurant designers, refrigeration experts, and even lighting technicians have all influenced the food-related decisions you've made today. And will make tomorrow. Maybe you've heard about the standard supermarket practice of putting common household items all the way at the back of the store so that you have to walk by lots of tempting and more expensive items to get your milk. That's a good example of the forces at hand to influence your built environment (their motivation is to make you stay longer in the store and spend more money, but it often leads to more crap food in your cart), but it's just the tip of the iceberg. Most of the attempts to influence you are out of range of your day-to-day radar. But I'm here to enlighten you and improve that radar!

The Science of Macro and Micro Built Environments

To appreciate how much is going on just outside your awareness when it comes to food decisions, you've got to know all about Brian Wansink, a former comedian turned professor (now at Cornell), researcher, and author who has done all the seminal studies of the ways in which our built environment impacts the food choices we make (yes, even the ones we're sure we're making of our own free will!).

When Professor Wansink first started thinking about why we eat too much, conventional wisdom about the relationship of eating to environment consisted of two main theories:

1. The *macro* environment drives most unhealthy behavior. That is, the combined impact of things like the number of parks in your neighborhood, your proximity to fast-food chains and cheap soda, and a lack of nutritional education was considered to be the chief negative influence on health and wellness. This became known as the "obese-o-genic" environment theory.

2. People always act rationally when their self-interest is at stake. Given the choice between something that is obviously really good for you and something that is obviously bad for you, most people will most often choose the thing that's good. This was kind of an evolutionary-theory-based line of thought, since our survival as a species depends on making smart and good-for-us decisions, right?

The obese-o-genic theory is clearly rational and true to a degree: it's true that more green spaces and fewer Golden

Arches near your home can have a positive impact (so long as you use the parks and don't go out of your way to find the Arches). And better food labeling and nutrition education in schools gives you the tools to understand the decisions you are making (but you have to *use* those tools).

But what about the second theory? It's kind of absurd. If it were always true, people wouldn't smoke cigarettes anymore. And they wouldn't text and drive. And they would consistently opt for veggies instead of French fries when offered the choice. And they'd always serve themselves a bowl of cut fruit instead of standing in the long line at the ice cream sundae bar.

A man ahead of his time, Professor Wansink looked around and could see that the conventional wisdom was at the very least incomplete, if not outright wrong. For starters, he could see what you and I do: people often *don't* act rationally. And he wondered if perhaps *micro* environmental cues would influence everyday decisions more than the macro ones (the big structural things that are less in our control).

To test whether people listen to their appetite or take their cues about eating from the way it's presented to them, he devised a sneaky experiment called the Soup Bowl Study. He brought sixty students into his lab/cafe for a free lunch, but what half of the diners didn't know was that the bowl of soup set before them was being continually refilled by a cleverly hidden system under the table. They were eating from a subtly bottomless soup bowl!

Guess what happened? People eating out of the bottomless soup bowl ate 73 percent more soup than those eating from an unrigged bowl. And those overeaters didn't report feeling any more full! How could they be full, they explained; they still had half a bowl of soup left to eat.

The lesson? We get full when we finish what's served; we eat with our eyes, not with our stomachs!

Need more proof? Professor Wansink has done many eye-opening experiments over the years. Here's another one: Do you think the shape of the glass you use affects how much you drink? Wansink gave eighty-nine adults who were eating breakfast either short or tall drinking glasses (different shape, but same volume capacity). He then gave them containers of juice and had them pour their own servings.

The finding: people poured 19 percent more juice in the short, wide glass (6.8 ounces) than in the tall glass (5.7 ounces). They mistakenly perceived that they had poured less into the wide glasses than into the tall glasses. Seventy-nine percent of the adults given the short, wide glasses underestimated how much they poured, as compared with 17 percent of those given tall glasses.

The more experiments he did, the more convinced Wansink became about one implication: when it comes to eating, small things make a huge difference.

In other words, maybe even more than things in our *macro* environment, it's the things in our *micro* environment that warp our ability to make good decisions. But the good news is that micro issues are ones you can control. You can't single-handedly convert a fast-food chain into a green park, but you *can* make micro changes!

More things I've learned from Brian Wansink and his amazing books:

- You will eat less if you transfer food from its packaging to a serving plate or bowl. The key is being able to see the size of your serving. So if you think you're saving yourself cleaning time by just eating directly out of that gallon of ice cream, think again. Go ahead and dirty that dish!

- What's on your kitchen counter has a direct correlation to the number on your scale: "If there's a box of cookies or bag of potato chips, occupants weighed nine pounds more than the norm. If cereal was visible, they weighed 21 lb. more. Any soft drink—even one can of diet cola—and they weighed 25 lb. more. If they had a fruit bowl, on the other hand, they weighed eight pounds less."

- When you serve white pasta on a white plate, you'll serve 18 percent more than you would if you used a colored plate. Break out your Fiestaware!

- Where you sit in a restaurant matters: you will eat more if you sit in a dark booth, near the TV, or near the bar. Ask the hostess to put you at a table away from the sports fans!

- And this one, which just floors me: you are 80 percent more likely to order vegetables if you sit near a window at a restaurant. As Wansink explained in an interview, "It could be that sitting next to a window cues the mind to freshness; in a back booth, it's out-of-control indulgence."

Reengineering Your Physical Environment

So how do we use all this scientific insight to fight weight gain and increase our individual chances for creating healthy habits? Obviously, understanding the forces that drive you to eat too much is key. Be aware of the tricks that the supermarket is playing and the ways in which lighting and plate choice and glass size influence your food decisions. That's the first step: awareness.

But then you can reengineer your own little world. Use your newfound understanding to create a world where making the healthy choice becomes easier and, eventually, unconscious.

Remember Danny Cahill? Joining a gym where he could enjoy a social network of like-minded "losers" was a critical first step, but even the most dedicated gym-rat can get sidetracked, and Danny soon discovered that he had to get his healthy lifestyle cues closer to home as well. He put a treadmill in front of his TV. "I made myself another deal: you want to watch TV, you go on the treadmill." (Note: this is also a good example of Habit 1—it's an *if/then* tactic!)

As he looked around his home, Danny started seeing other things he could do to change his micro built environment. "I needed that feeling of changing for the better, and I realized I had to make things look different from the way things looked when I was fat. I put in a new floor. I have two grills outside the door now. My refrigerator is even different!" Danny now maintains a healthy 240 pounds.

OH, BEHAVE!

Oh, the dreaded buffet—whether it's the all-you-can-eat one at your favorite restaurant or the office party, we're all kind of afraid of it. Or, better put: we're afraid of losing our control around it! Fear no more. Brian Wansink has studied how *thin* people behave around buffets (yes, it *is* possible to behave around a buffet!). Here is what his research shows:

- Thin people tend to sit about sixteen feet farther from food than heavy people.
- Thin people are three times as likely to face away from food.
- Seventy-one percent of thin people scout the food, walking around before picking up a plate.

Danny was consciously acting on an important part of Brian Wansink's insight: engineering small visual cues—at home and away—can bring about big changes. That's why I want you to pay special attention to the Habit Homework below. Habit 1 got you thinking about contingency planning for new behavior. Habit 2 armed you with a pushback plan to guard against negative thinking and defeatism. Now you've got to get your house in order to make healthy habits automatic—literally part of your life!

HABIT HOMEWORK

Change the architecture of your social environment:

- Make a list of the things you do that you know are unhealthy and another list of things you consider to be supportive of your thin maintenance or goals. Now write down the names of the people with whom you most often engage in each kind of behavior. See a pattern emerging? That awareness is half the battle.

- Now that you have identified the people who are not so good for you (in the skinny sense), brainstorm how you can either change the dynamic of the relationship or start to spend more time with people with whom you're more likely to do healthy, Skinny Habits– supporting things. Maybe suggest to your afternoon cookie run buddy that you walk instead of drive from now on. Or better yet, that you swap the cookie for coffee instead.

- Reconsider the who/what/when of your food-shopping routine. Do you shop with someone (your sugar-loving kid, perhaps?) who leads you down the processed-foods aisle every time? Do you shop after work toward the end of the week when you're inevitably tired and hungry (and needing to "treat yourself" to something that rewards all your hard work)? How about leaving Junior at home next time and shopping after eating a good breakfast on Saturday? I'll bet you can make healthier decisions about what goes home with you if you don't have your usual cues and distractions.

- If you don't already have a workout group or buddy, make a list of people you know who might be interested. Put their phone numbers next to their names. Call at least one person on that list within one week of reading this book.
- Make a date to get together for some kind of physical exertion: walk the dog together, go for a hike, go to that crazy spin class you've been afraid to try alone.
- If you already have a workout group or buddy, but you've been less than consistent in getting together, pick one member of the group as your workout sponsor and make a deal with him or her: I'll call you the night before if I can't make it. No surprise cancellations. (This is another if/then contingency plan!)

Change the architecture of your built environment:

- Walk around your home and try to identify every possible cue or "fat trap," as Professor Wansink calls them, in the place. You're looking for the obvious things that either trigger fat habits behavior or hinder Skinny Habits behavior: the cabinet filled with sugary treats, the beer fridge within reach of your reclining chair, your reclining chair (!), the way your treadmill is hidden under your dry-cleaning pile. And you're looking for the not-so-immediately obvious: the massive coffee mugs that more often than not are filled with hot cocoa and *not* coffee, the collapsible trays that make it easy to eat in front of the TV, the really disorganized workout-clothes drawer.

- Walk around your office and do the same kind of inventory: note where the vending machines are and how you've made them a stop on your regular route to the bathroom. Don't have vending machines at work? I'll bet there's someone in the office who has a dangerously delicious bowl of candy on their desk, and I'd be willing to bet that you just *happen* to pass that desk regularly.

- Now that you've identified the things that trip you up or stand in your way at home and at work, brainstorm ways to reengineer your patterns in both places. You can start by cleaning out that snack cabinet—toss out the junk food and stock up on healthier snacks. Move on to setting up your kitchen or dining room to make it conducive to use (or make the couch in front of the TV *less* conducive). Maybe put out some candles? Cloth napkins? Or how about just making sure the table is cleared off and clean?! If your recliner has your butt print on it, consider giving it away. Organize that workout-clothes drawer so you don't have any excuses not to dip into it. Go one step further and lay a workout outfit at the foot of your bed so that you have to make an active decision *not* to put it on in the morning!

- Apply your if/then muscles to your reengineering efforts. "If Carol wants to go to the food trucks for dumplings, I'll suggest we go the other way around the block and head toward the farmer's market. And if Carol convinces me to go to the trucks anyway, I'll get a small order of the veggie dumplings instead of the large pork ones!"

At Home

Don't get overwhelmed by this habit. You don't have to do everything at once! Here are a few simple things you can do today. They'll get you on your way to creating a fitter environment for yourself. Feel free to innovate!

- Grab a big trash basket and fill it with any and all food items that you and your family should never eat. You know.
- Put your sports bra, running shoes, and shorts next to your bed. (Men can forgo the bra unless required.)
- Set your alarm clock on "loud" and put it in another room so you have to get up to shut it off before deciding to go back to sleep rather than go for your morning walk.
- Buy an inexpensive guide to the caloric content of all food; make sure it covers all convenience foods. Put one copy in your car and one copy in the kitchen.
- Read the above book—any part of it!—for *just five minutes* before you go grocery shopping.

Away from Home

- Buy some apples and put them in a bowl on your desk at work.
- Put a blank calendar next to your desk; make a black checkmark on it every day you exercise.
- Do an online search of healthy restaurants near work. Print out a list and pin it next to your calendar.
- If you work for a large (or progressive enough) company, check out what fitness benefits it offers. You can usually find this information easily and quickly through your human resources department.
- Put a pair of running shoes and an absorbent towel in your desk drawer.

six

HABIT 4:
CHALLENGE YOURSELF

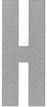ere's a little good news: this Skinny Habit doesn't ask anything of you *immediately*. As in, you don't have to do something specific right this minute, today, or even this week. The Habit Homework at the end of the chapter falls more in the "brainstorm, daydream, and consider making plans" realm than "do these five things now." Eventually you're going to have to attend to this habit, though. Because my saying "come back to it when you can" or "think about this and act on it when you're inspired" *absolutely does not* mean that this is an *optional* Skinny Habit! Hell no!

And do you know what I'm guessing? Making this habit part of your life might actually be the most fun you've had all year.

TOXIC BOREDOM

Have you ever had to fill out a questionnaire that asked you to list your hobbies? Maybe for a job interview? Why the heck does a prospective employer care what you do in your nonworking time? Simple: they want to assess if you're a one-dimensional bore or if you'd bring some knowledge and experiences that could contribute to the office morale and/or inspire others.

Or maybe you had to do this at the doctor's office. The last time I had my annual physical, the doctor's pre-exam paperwork included answering the question "What are your hobbies?" I understood why that question was there: doctors know that having outside interests keeps you lively, alive, engaged in life; they are good defenses against depression. The absence of them is a red flag.

I'm not your employer and I'm not your doctor, but do you know what I almost always see as a common factor in the lives of the people I coach through weight loss? Regardless of the person's gender, their educational background, their socioeconomic status, their age, or where they live, what almost all chronically overweight or obese people have in common is some form of boredom.

No matter the trigger or the reason for your boredom, no matter how obvious it is that you're experiencing it, if you have a weight problem, I'm going to bet you also have boredom issues! And any amount of boredom is a bad thing. To your soul, boredom is toxic. To your body, ditto. Boredom leaves you tired, unengaged, isolated, purposeless, self-loathing, and, yes, really boring. All things that lead to eating too much and moving too little.

Sometimes the boredom in the people I coach is obvious—even to them. They have limited interests and don't really feel deeply about any one thing they spend their time doing. That sort of blah feeling has spilled over into their health and they've become overweight. It's not that they are disinterested in their health (if that were the case, they wouldn't have sought me out), but their general malaise has made them lazy about it.

More often, the boredom is much less obvious because these people are busier than they can possibly articulate ("Bob, I'm too busy to tell you how busy I am!") and wouldn't think to describe themselves as bored at all. But scratch the surface of their reality and it turns out that they are busy with a job that doesn't really inspire them or dealing with a relationship that is just so-so. Or maybe they are pretty happy (if tired) juggling a thousand responsibilities—parenting, working, carpooling, grocery shopping, helping their aging parents, fixing the house—but their responsibilities have become a grind. They may be busy but they are not busy doing anything *that gives them joy or satisfaction*. So, actually, although some of the multitude of responsibilities are inspiring and invigorating (raising kids surely gives life meaning), these people aren't reserving time on that busy, busy calendar for something all their own. The bottom line: being busy for busy-ness' sake is its own form of boredom. If

There are lots of semibored people out there who *do not* have a weight problem. What distinguishes them from you? They have managed to carve out just a little bit of time for something they *do* love, or for a cause larger than themselves. They have endless responsibilities too, but every now and then they devote some time to something other than their to-do list; they do something purely for the joy and challenge of it. And that joy permeates their life in ways that are undeniably healthy. And, ultimately, slimming!

you have endless responsibilities and never sit down and focus on the things you might have once dreamed of doing with your life, if you are so darn busy that you can't, well, see the forest for the trees, you've become a busy bore!

Know anyone like that?

YOUR BRAIN ON A CHALLENGE

If you look across the many studies of people who maintain mental agility, flexibility, and strength, you'll quickly discover that learning—and the mental challenge that comes with it—sits at the center of healthy brain regimens. Remember our discussion of memory formation back in Chapter 2? Many of the same physical processes are at play here as well. *Repeated sensory experience enlarges memory pathways, and bigger memory paths seem to make for a healthier, more agile brain*—the kind we increasingly need in the fast-moving, ever-changing world around us. The kind we need to change habits.

So, what's the antidote to boredom? This is actually very simple: you need to light a fire; you need to consistently, and positively, stimulate your brain. You need to use your creative juices, learn something new, be challenged! If you think about it, it's challenge that helps build many of the most important qualities we value in this fast-changing world: mental agility, flexibility, the ability to learn quickly, and, importantly for your weight-loss goals, to recover from setback. If you want to cast it all in fitness terms: you can't get a healthy brain without a healthy challenge.

No two ways about it: challenge is a key element of cognitive health. For decades scientists believed that the brain stopped forming new connections after about age thirty-five; brain development was thought to be only for the young. But about ten years ago all of that changed as new brain-imaging techniques (called fMRI, or functional MRI) revealed that older brains are able to regenerate brain cells and reconnect them, too. This was evidence of something that scientists didn't really know was applicable to adult brains: neuroplasticity, the ability of our noggins to grow new internal connections. This means that pathways that carry signals for everything from memory to reading to athletic coordination—all of which naturally atrophy as we age—can be strengthened later in life!

Let's first take up mental challenge—things like learning the guitar (my new thing!) or reading something difficult. These are activities that *disturb your usual routines and*

> Being bored is *very* different from being able to relax and do nothing. Being bored is the absence of interest instead of the act of pressing the pause button, which is what relaxation and rest amount to. Being bored is a vacuum—it sucks the life out of you. Being able to rest and relax is a skill that we'll turn into a habit for you in the next chapter.

require extra effort. The brain then reacts to the challenge by producing all kinds of chemicals. These molecules seem to induce new mental capacities as well as maintain old ones. Anyone trying to form new habits needs exactly such strengths.

What happens when I struggle over the finger placement for a certain chord? (And boy do I struggle!) Or when I strain to read a new piece of music? All those notes and tempo instructions sometimes seem to float all over the page while I try to follow along! I need to focus pretty intently to master a new piece. I get so wrapped up in the effort that sometimes hours will go by without my even knowing it. And sometimes I haven't made too much progress on the piece. Have I wasted those precious hours? Has my single-minded focus stunted my brain development for that "lost" time?

Absolutely not. All that effort at hand-eye coordination and that focus on tone, pitch, and timing has a big mental payoff.

In 2012, a group of researchers at Emory University

There are all kinds of devices and software programs on the market that promise to challenge and improve your mental agility (though any that claim they will "prevent" Alzheimer's or Parkinson's disease are not credible!). Try these if they appeal to you. But simply reading a book (that might require you to look up words you don't know) or doing a complicated puzzle that demands time and focus are great options, too. Or, like me, learn a musical instrument. Although it is still unclear just how much brain training transfers to other activities, I'm convinced that these small things add up.

studying the effect of intensive training on the aging adult brain did a groundbreaking experiment. They were particularly interested in studying the arcuate fasciculus (Latin for "curved bundle"), a bundle of neurological connections in the brain involved in vision, reaction time, and emotional processing. They wanted to see how those areas of the brain were impacted by the study and practice of a musical instrument.

They scanned one group of adults who practiced some musical task on a regular basis. They did the same for nonmusicians of the same age and health status. The results surprised even the most skeptical of the scholars. The nonmusicians showed predictable declines in volume of the arcuate fasciculus. The musicians, on the other hand, showed no such degeneration. The finding seemed to reinforce previous work showing that musicians also had greater gray matter in portions of the brain associated with reasoning and logic. They concluded: "Musicians appear to be less susceptible to age-related degenerations in the brain, presumably as a result of their daily musical activities."

What about other kinds of learning activities, like certain sports and creative endeavors? Yes! In a 2008 report, researchers reported the results of another scanning study. In this one, they investigated what must have been a fun subject: what changes would happen in the gray matter of sixty-year-olds who were exposed to intense training in . . . wait for it . . . juggling! Specifically, "three-ball cascade juggling" (the kind your Uncle Joe breaks out after he's had a few drinks on Thanksgiving). The finding: sixty-year-olds were not only able to learn the techniques to juggle, they also showed gray matter increases in key learning, motivation, and pleasure regions of the brain. Conclusion: "These findings suggest the potential value of plasticity-based training in preserving brain functions in the elderly."

But maybe you're young and not yet concerned with cognitive decline. You think that's many, many years in the future. I hope that for you too, but even if you're young, the advice is relevant: challenging yourself can widen your neural pathways and allow them to accommodate new habits. It's a way to build new strengths. Old or young.

Researchers have since discovered all kinds of links between mental health and novel learning experiences—again, things that challenge you. Hobbies, from fast-action sports like Ping-Pong to things like knitting, sewing, and . . . quilting!

Yes, even quilting seems to have a profound effect on brain health. Participants in a community study of quilters in 2012 reported that the creative process "captivated" them, distracted them, and gave them an experience not unlike the "flow" that great athletes always talk about. In fact, the psychological benefits from "flow" lasted after participants had stopped quilting. Check out what they said:

> [Quilting] just puts it [anxieties] into a different perspective, you are viewing it in a different light . . . you are doing something that you are enjoying . . . are a bit lighter in what you are thinking . . . when you come away from it [quilting] you are not in the same mood.

Not in the same mood. Doing something you are enjoying. A bit lighter in what you are thinking. Oh my goodness, and flow too? All good. Do you need more evidence that getting off the couch and into a new hobby will be a great defense—a kind of Kryptonite you can hold up against weight gain? Do you already want to eat less and move around a little more just by thinking about the fun you could be having?

FLOW THROUGH SERVICE

Developing a hobby isn't the only way of stimulating your brain, of improving your neuroplasticity, of becoming less bored and boring. The key is feeling passion for something— but that something doesn't have to be learning a new instrument or language, or doing crossword puzzles or quilting or juggling. You might develop a passion for some kind of service to others, and that too has the same kind of neurological benefit. And, of course, the same kind of trickle-down Kryptonite effect on weight gain!

One of the more gratifying aspects of my job is that I get to check in with clients and contestants and see what they've been doing since they lost their weight. One of the more interesting—and wonderful—things that keeps coming up is service: putting in effort and time helping others.

Danny Cahill, the reengineering mastermind we met earlier, tells the story of being inspired to serve and reach out to others by an email he received from a seven-year-old boy in Brazil named Bernardo. Bernardo had seen Danny—and followed his weight-loss struggle—on TV and was writing to thank Danny for inspiration and to ask for an autographed picture. A follow-up email from Bernardo's father explained that Bernardo had been born prematurely and had been in the ICU for 101 days thereafter. Doctors said he wouldn't have the mobility of normal children and would even have severe learning disabilities. When he saw Danny's story on the show, his father explained, Bernardo had said, "Father, my friend Danny is just like me; he doesn't give up easily. When I grow up I want to spread the message he spreads that you can do anything no matter your circumstance."

Danny was touched by Bernardo's story. "So here's this little guy from Brazil. He's sick, but he's writing me to ask for a photo so he can stay inspired. That got me! I realized it's not just all about me now. It's about other people and paying it forward." Danny took that revelation and ran with it. In addition to the boot camp–style workout class that he now teaches, Danny has written two books and gives motivational speeches all around the world.

As Danny's experience shows, serving others and giving to others is not about writing a check to your favorite charity. I encourage you to do that *too,* but in order to get the emotional benefit of giving to others, you need to show up, you need to engage. And keep showing up and engaging. If you can manage to combine a desire to give back and to inspire others with your "day job," so much the better!

HABIT HOMEWORK

Pretend I'm interviewing you. I want you to write down what your hobbies and interests are. Feel free to say that your kids are your "outside interest" or that cooking for your family is a hobby. Those may be true statements. But you also need to come up with at least one not-otherwise-linked-to-your-responsibilities list. If you can come up with that one thing—fishing, hiking, playing the flute, raising chickens, whatever!—that's excellent news. Now you need to make some time for that enjoyable activity, because chances are you've been giving it short shrift lately.

If you've got nothing—nothing outside of your regular routine to pique your interest—try this: Think back to when you were younger. Can you remember what you wanted to be when you grew up? Or "where you wanted to

Having trouble coming up with a way to serve others? Do any of these ideas inspire you?

Serve Others

- Serve food at your local food bank (feedingamerica.org).
- Walk rescue dogs at your local dog shelter (petfinder.com).
- Help veterans in need (volunteer.va.gov).
- Read to children at your local school.
- Join an advocacy group and fight for a cause you believe in.
- Teach a class (on whatever you know) at your local senior home.
- Train your dog to be a therapy dog, and visit clinics and hospitals.
- Visit an elderly neighbor and offer to help in any way that's needed.
- Start a community garden.
- Check out online volunteer coordination sites—both local ones and national ones like volunteermatch.org or createthegood.org—and get inspired!

Challenge Yourself

- Learn a musical instrument.
- Join a knitting group.
- Sign up for a community art class.
- Learn a new language.
- Grow vegetables.
- Learn to juggle.

- Find a table tennis club.
- Learn self-defense.
- Audition for community theater.
- Take a salsa dance class.

be in ten years" when you graduated from college? The sky was the limit, right? So what did you want to do with your life then?

Now, think of ways you might be able to bridge the gap . . . what small things might you be able to do now that could reinvigorate those youthful dreams?

For instance: Did you want to travel around the world? Is there some way you can bring a more global view into your life without having to actually get on a plane? Maybe you can take a cooking class (Chinese, Italian, French), host an exchange student, or get involved in a charity that raises money and collects supplies for people in need abroad. Can you take a class to learn one of the languages you'd hoped to have mastered by now?

What about trying to learn an instrument? You may not ever become the rock star you imagined you'd be back when you were young, but by this time next year you *could be* the person who entertains the crowd at the holiday party by whipping out that guitar or sitting down at the piano!

seven

HABIT 5:
REST FOR SUCCESS

You probably know that I have a thing for . . . water. Drinking enough of it every day is Rule 1 of *The Skinny Rules*. You just can't lose weight and keep it off if you don't drink your water.

Rule 19 of *Skinny Rules* covered another essential "ingredient" for successful weight loss: sleep. Like water, it's a wellspring of health. And like water, no one seems to get enough. But unlike drinking a glass of water when you start to get thirsty, getting "enough" sleep isn't a quick proposition. The recommended amount of sleep is six to nine hours! Not quick at all. And then of course there's the issue of *getting to sleep* even when you make the time in your schedule for the needed allotment. Too often you get yourself into bed "on time," intending to give yourself a full night's worth, but you just can't seem to nod off. All of

Sleep is an essential ingredient in overall health and in your ability to lose weight. Yet so far the scientific search for a good sleeping pill has yielded very little. There are sleeping medications that will make you prone to amnesia, obesity, hallucinations, and car crashes if you're not careful. One even makes everything taste like aluminum! But there is nothing that reliably gets you through the sleep cycles required for body and mind repair and restoration. Looks like you're going to have to get it the old-fashioned way: naturally.

which is why so many people tell me that Rule 19 is one they just can't quite master.

So what's the secret? What's the behavior that thin people know and do that you need to embrace? It's not only that healthily thin people generally tend to respect their need for sleep more than you might, and it's not only that they don't take their phones to bed with them (please stop doing that and other things listed on page 120!). No, it's more than that. It's this: *thin people know how to rest and relax.* Not only do they get more rest (sleep), but they can shut their minds "off" and get to sleep more quickly and stay asleep longer when they allot the time for it.

THE RHYTHM OF THE NIGHT

No, not that dance tune!

I'm talking about your circadian rhythm, your internal

"sleep clock." The term *circadian* comes from the Latin words *circa,* which means "approximately," and *diem,* which means "day." Which makes sense, because your circadian rhythm ticks along over the course of about twenty-four hours, starting over each new day. Although your circadian rhythm is an innate, or built-in, thing, it takes its cues from your environment. Like, say, night and day! Light cues you to wake up (or stay awake). Darkness cues sleep. Alter the light you're exposed to and your circadian rhythm gets out of whack. Like when you put the clock forward or back at daylight savings. Or travel across time zones.

Of course, there are other things that screw up your circadian rhythm, things that cue you to stay awake when you want to sleep. Alcohol can mess with your system in all kinds of ways, but the disorientation that comes from drinking too much of it can numb you to your circadian rhythm (until you just pass out, whether it's night or day!). Computer and phone screens emit a kind of light that can keep you awake.

And then there's the big daddy of sleep disruption: your *daytime* rhythm. If you are crazy-busy and stressed out, your internal physiological balance is affected (more on your body's response to stress shortly), and your sleep-wake cycle can get way out of whack as a result. All around not good.

YOUR BRAIN AND BODY ON A DECENT NIGHT'S SLEEP

When you sleep well, you give your body a chance to grow, repair, and recover from your daily demands. Think of it this way: your day-to-day life—from breathing and moving to talking and exercising—*takes* from you. Sleep *gives back*. A whole host of bodily activities happen during good sleep: your blood pressure goes down, your vital organs produce more beneficial hormones (mainly growth hormone and testosterone), your immune system gets a boost, and specialized cells sweep the brain of waste products.

So what constitutes *decent,* anyway? For starters, your six to nine hours (for me, personally, I've found that I function best on eight hours) should be uninterrupted, consecutive. You can't get four hours in the early evening, wake up for five, then get a handful more before dawn and hope to reap the health (and sanity) benefits of the total number of hours you strung together. Why? Again: rhythm.

When you sleep, you are actually cycling through phases of different quality sleep, and you've got to stay asleep for a while to get to the really good stuff! Think of it as spiraling happily down into rest, with periodic phases of crazy dreaming and brain wackiness. You go from light sleep to deeper, to deepest. Then you pop "up" into that dreaming, hallucination phase, then light, deeper, deepest all over again. I'll break it down:

For the first five to ten minutes of shut-eye (when you are asleep as opposed to just lying there wishing you were), you are in very light sleep. You might twitch or feel like you're falling if you're aware of your surroundings at all. This is a non-rapid-eye movement phase (n-REM).

The second phase of deeper sleep lasts about twenty minutes. It's during this time that your heart rate slows and your body temperature goes down. This is also an n-REM phase.

The third phase is often called "delta sleep" because of the slow brain waves (delta waves) that occur. You're basically out like a light at this point—you aren't going to be very responsive to noises and you are deeply asleep. Your body really needs to get to this point in the sleep cycle—this is the physically restorative and peaceful sleep you need to recover from the day. But this peaceful deep sleep doesn't last long. It tends to last five to ten minutes, and then you cycle back to that second phase again, before you head off to . . .

Rapid-eye-movement sleep: REM. You have a lot of brain activity during REM sleep. That doesn't mean you aren't resting and repairing, but your brain has sort of come back online. This is when you dream. But though your brain is active, your body is not. Your muscles are really relaxed, so relaxed that your "voluntary" muscles—the ones you have to be conscious to move as opposed to, say, your heart, which goes on beating even if you're unconscious—are actually paralyzed!

Like that first spurt of n-REM sleep, this first experience of REM might not last too long, but as your body cycles back up to the second n-REM phase (and then back to REM, and so on), each segment tends to get longer.

Bottom line: the longer you stay asleep, the longer you get in that really restorative place. If you interrupt your sleep (noises, lights, phone calls or incoming email pings, stressful list making in the middle of the night), you have to start from the top each time you fall back asleep, which means you'll limit the length of the stretches in that really happy place.

YOUR BODY AND BRAIN ON A LACK OF SLEEP

Lack of sleep—particularly the right kind of sleep I've described above—has been linked to a wide range of modern chronic diseases. Though we don't know exactly *how* sleep deprivation drives illness, the list of sleep-related disease is long and ever-growing. If you don't get enough sleep, your risk for heart disease, diabetes, and immune deficiency skyrockets. Memory, reaction time, and the ability to focus plummet. Memory lapses and inability to focus aren't good things for one's habit formation, that's for sure.

Researchers have known for years that people who sleep less than five or six hours a night have a higher risk of being overweight, and they are now looking into why that is. Scientific studies are starting to shed light on what many of us experience, firsthand, on a regular basis!

The Brain and Your Belly

A recent study at the University of California, Berkeley, investigated the impact of sleep deprivation on the brain. After just one night of inadequate sleep, pronounced changes were seen in the way the subjects' brains responded to calorie-dense junk food. The researchers saw *increased* activity in the part of the brain associated with the motivation to eat, and *decreased* activity in the frontal cortex—the part of your brain responsible for weighing up consequences and making rational decisions. Now *that's* what I call a high-risk combo for anyone trying to live the skinny life!

Metabolism and Eating Habits

Sleep researchers from the University of Colorado conducted a small study to investigate the effects of sleep patterns on metabolism and eating habits. Half the people in the group were allowed nine hours of shut-eye, while the other half were only allowed to sleep up to five hours. Even though the sleep-deprived subjects showed an increase in metabolism (possibly due to more time spent moving around), they ate far more than the well-rested subjects (more time to eat, after all!) and gained an average of about two pounds after just one week of inadequate sleep! Not surprisingly, they ate way too many carbohydrates and ate more after dinner.

Hormones

Other studies on the metabolic consequences of sleep deprivation have looked at hormonal changes in sleep-deprived subjects. The hormones leptin and ghrelin are involved with appetite regulation and energy expenditure. Leptin is the "satiety" hormone. It dampens your appetite and tells you that you are full, and it increases your energy output. Ghrelin—the "hunger" hormone—does the opposite. Research has shown that inadequate sleep is associated with lower levels of leptin and higher levels of ghrelin in the blood, which—guess what?—makes us want to eat more and exercise less!

Stress Levels

Some studies have shown an increase in cortisol levels—the stress-response hormone—in subjects who are sleep-deprived. Higher cortisol levels encourage the body to store more fat and make the body more inclined to use muscle tissue as a source of energy. If that sounds like a dodgy combination, it is! Studies suggest that sleep-deprived people are more likely to gain fat and lose muscle than their well-rested counterparts.

The Biology of Fat Cells

A small study carried out at the University of Chicago showed that sleep deprivation alters the biology of fat cells. Researchers monitored the changes that occurred in subjects who moved from eight and a half hours of sleep a night to only four and a half hours. After just four nights of sleep deprivation, the subjects' fat cells showed decreased sensitivity to insulin, a metabolic change that has been linked to obesity and diabetes.

So, in summary, if you are . . .

- Craving junk food
- Unable to rationally resist aforementioned junk food
- Feeling too lethargic to work out
- Unable to feel full
- Feeling stressed
- Gaining weight

... then before you start beating yourself over the head for being a Skinny Rules dropout, ask yourself this one simple question: Am I getting enough sleep?

If the answer is no, then the odds are stacked against you. Do yourself—and your waistline—a favor. Make sure you are getting enough zzz's, and sleep your way to a better body.

YOUR BODY AND BRAIN ON STRESS— AND RELAXATION

Okay, you believe me now: you need to get more sleep. But try as you might, you just can't do it. You can't seem to turn your mind "off" at night in order to get to sleep in the first place! That's most often because of stress.

You've likely heard of the fight-or-flight response. It's also known as the "stress response." Whatever you call it, it refers to the body's response to a perceived threat. The threat could be real—a loose zoo animal! A tornado! A mugger! Or it might be less immediate but no less anger- or fear-inducing: a looming deadline at work, a terrible traffic jam on the highway, an argument with your spouse, or just a really *long* to-do list (and not enough time to do even half of it). Simply put: either you feel compelled to run *at* the problem (lash out at it) or you want to turn tail and run *away* (flight mode). You feel anxiety when you're in fight mode, and in flight mode, depression. You experience an increase in heart rate, breathing rate, blood pressure, and body temperature. You sweat.

When we are in fight-or-flight mode, blood flow is channeled away from the digestive system and poured into muscles so that we are ready to either tackle the perceived threat or run for our lives. This diversion affects everything from our saliva glands (dry mouth syndrome) to our stomach (nausea/constipation) and is supposed to be only temporary. In the short term, survival is more important than digestion.

But many of us remain in a state of high alert, juggling responsibilities and trying to keep up with the hectic pace of our lives. Chronic stress causes many health problems, so it is not surprising that it is notorious for causing a whole host of digestive issues. Studies have also shown a link between chronic stress and obesity—through direct mechanisms like increasing appetite and food intake as well as indirect mechanisms like decreasing sleep and exercise. Of course decreased sleep—as we talked about above—also has an impact on those direct mechanisms, like food intake!

So, if the fight-or-flight response is like pressing the gas pedal in your car, where are the brakes?

What I like to call the rest-and-digest response, also known as the "relaxation response," is the exact opposite of fight-or-flight. It is the physiological response that is designed to calm your whole system and restore balance after the aforementioned danger has passed.

Being able to turn on the "relaxation response" is not only good for our minds, it is good for our waistlines, and it literally allows our bodies to "rest and digest." In this state, everything is brought back to order, and all of our systems are given the blood supply they need to function properly. This is the state in which optimum healing and digestion occur.

RELAX, MAN

So, which way to the brake pedal?

Dr. Herbert Benson, director emeritus of the Benson-Henry Institute for Mind Body Medicine at Massachusetts General Hospital and Mind Body Medicine Professor of Medicine at Harvard Medical School, coined the term "the relaxation response." He wrote a bestselling book by the same name in 1975. Dr. Benson has spent much of his forty-plus-year medical career researching ways to prompt the relaxation response in order to counter the damaging effects of stress. Among his top recommendations? Mindfulness meditation, yoga, and belly breathing. Let's tackle these one at a time:

Mindfulness

Mindfulness meditation grew out of Buddhism as practiced in India. It's one of the simplest forms of meditation there is:

you sit, comfortably and quietly, eyes closed, and focus on your breath. If you're like everyone else, your mind will immediately start wandering. Don't worry. Don't judge yourself. Just return to a focus on your breath. Try it for about ten minutes at first. Don't beat yourself up if you can't stay focused on the in and out of your breath the whole time. The point is to keep going back to a focus on your breath. And don't be surprised if this intense focus gets you breathing funny! As you practice you'll connect more deeply with your breathing; you'll slowly breathe easier. And you'll disconnect from the problems, emotions, and obstacles that trip up your daily life. You'll be able to see them for what they are. It's almost like getting a bird's-eye view of your own life!

Until recently, we didn't have any way to understand how mindfulness works. Now, with new brain-scanning technologies, we can zero in on what parts of the brain get activated during meditation. An interesting experiment was conducted at the University of Utah recently. Researchers had fourteen meditators enter a sophisticated scanning device and begin breath-focused meditation. The participants were instructed to press a button in front of them when their mind wandered and they lost focus. An analysis showed something amazing (and not anticipated) during focused meditation. Specific areas of the brain—including our friend the basal ganglia—were linked to specific changes: improvements in attention, increased bodily sensations, and decreased negative self-thoughts, anxiety, and rumination. All three, especially reduced anxiety and negative self-thoughts, were linked to relaxation, improved mood, and better sleep. Other studies have demonstrated benefits for insomniacs, sufferers of OCD, and depressives.

Yoga

Unless you've been hibernating in an igloo somewhere for the last decade or so, you likely know that yoga has taken off in this country. It's become an industry in itself, with pricey instructors, clothes, retreats, and even yoga competitions (which is kind of weird if you think about it!). But you don't need to go all yogi to get the relaxation (and brain) benefits of a few simple positions.

Yoga also originated in India. In Sanskrit it means "yoking" of body and mind, but for our purposes it mainly means *listening*—paying attention to what's in front of you *right now*. That's important to keep in mind. The swamis and other holy men who first developed it 2,700 years ago mainly had one thing in mind: teaching your body and mind to escape the attachments of everyday life, attachments like pride and greed and ego and desire. In the twentieth century, some of yoga's more adventuresome advocates came to the United States, where the practice evolved to accommodate the more practical concerns of modern life: anxiety, stress, ambition, and attachment to material things, including money. From there it evolved into today's most popular form, hatha yoga, a series of poses (called asanas) and breathing practices (known as pranayama).

True to our scientific orientation, we Westerners soon

THE BENEFITS OF LAVENDER OIL

Blissed-out yoga teachers sometimes waft lavender oil around the room at the end of class. They offer to dab it on your temples to help you relax. Lavender-scented beauty products jump off the shelves at you, claiming to soothe your skin and transport you to instant calm. Maybe your new workout partner douses herself in the stuff as she leaves the gym and heads off to work! There seems to be a whole tribe of lavender oil peddlers out there who are going misty-eyed at the mere mention of it. Sure it smells nice, but does it really work?

Well, if your personal experience of lavender oil is not enough to convince you of the benefits, consider this extract, taken from a multicenter, double-blind, randomized study conducted in Germany in 2009, comparing a lavender oil preparation called silexan to the benzodiazepine lorazepam (Ativan) as a treatment for generalized anxiety disorder (GAD): "In conclusion, our results demonstrate that silexan is as effective as lorazepam in adults with GAD. The safety of silexan was also demonstrated. Since lavender oil showed no sedative effects in our study and has no potential for drug abuse, silexan appears to be an effective and well tolerated alternative to benzodiazepines for amelioration of generalized anxiety."

Being rested and staying calm is an important part of staying skinny! So do as the yogis do. Dab a little lavender oil on your wrists, put a few drops in your bath, and consider treating yourself to a lavender-scented eye pillow. You deserve it!

began demanding proof that yoga "works." That led the National Institutes of Health and other serious research institutions around the world to conduct clinical trials, scrutinizing yoga's principal therapeutic claims, its antistress properties among them.

In 2006, a group of researchers at the University of Duisburg-Essen, in Germany, recruited twenty-four women to participate in a three-month study of hatha yoga. All of them were self-described as "emotionally distressed" at the outset. Each took a series of standardized tests that measure stress-related problems and stress hormones. Half of the group received two sessions a week of hatha yoga instruction; the other half did not.

At the end of the study, researchers again measured the stress indicators. In the yoga group, there were "pronounced and significant" improvements in just about every area. Patients reported big drops in anxiety, increases in well-being and vigor, and improvements in fatigue and depression. Subjects with chronic headaches and back pain got relief.

And there's more! One of the hormones that the researchers measured before and after the study was cortisol. The yoga group showed a large drop in cortisol levels. They also reported significant decreases in mental, emotional, and physical distress. A number of other studies undertaken since have reported similar results. One report even showed increases in growth hormone, associated with heart health, muscle increases, and cognitive improvements.

All that and cool workout clothes too?! I know, awesome! In the Habit Homework section below, you'll find the six yoga poses I want you to learn. Only six, and as you'll see, these poses don't require standing on your head! These are *super* easy, people. If you didn't know they were yoga poses, you might just call them . . . stretching!

Belly Breathing

Yoga instructors refer to "belly breathing" as a way to enter a restful state. But what the heck does it mean?

"Belly breathing" is the act of taking a deep breath through your nose and filling your lungs until your lower belly gently rises. Poetic license aside, we are not actually breathing into our bellies (as in through our belly buttons!). We are breathing fully and completely into our lungs, which, in turn, causes the diaphragm to drop down and press against your abdominal organs in order to make room for your expanding lungs to fill with air.

Whether you prefer poetic license or actual anatomy, the results are the same. There's no doubt about it—deep "belly breathing" is a powerful tonic for your whole system and a great way to prepare for sleep.

Many of us spend a lot of the day taking short, shallow "chest" breaths that are not only a *result* of stress, they *increase* stress. How's that for a double whammy? A pattern of tense, shallow breathing over time, caused by chronic stress and anxiety, deprives the body of oxygen, compromises the immune system, and taxes the nervous system.

Making a conscious switch to belly breathing is a great technique for literally slowing down your heart rate and sending a signal to your nervous system that it is time to unwind. Belly breathing also encourages full oxygen exchange—the healthy trade of incoming oxygen for outgoing carbon dioxide—and can help to lower or stabilize blood pressure.

Belly breathing is simple. Here's what you do: Lie on your back with your knees bent and your feet flat on the floor. Place your palms flat on your belly, just below your navel. Begin to inhale slowly and deeply, and allow your belly to gently rise up into your hands. As you slowly release your exhale, allow your belly to soften back toward the floor.

For an extra calming effect, see if you can make your exhales a little longer than your inhales by silently counting the length of your breath. For example, if you inhale for four counts, see if you can exhale for five or six counts, or longer. Find a rhythm that is comfortable for you.

CLEAN SLEEP

Yes, you should launder your sheets and bedding with some regularity, but this isn't a book about how to not be a slob and how to get dates!

Sleep hygiene refers to the routines you create around sleep (to support it) and the things you do and don't do to protect it. Healthily thin people know this intuitively. As much as possible, they do the following things, and you should too:

Do:

- Go to bed and get up at the same time each day.
- Establish a bedtime routine, such as a warm bath, reading, and a few yoga poses before lights out.
- Keep the temperature in your bedroom comfortable, or a little cool.
- Keep your feet warm. Wear socks if need be.
- Use comfortable bedding.
- Ensure that your bedroom is quiet and dark at night.
- Use your bed only for sleep and sex. No emailing, checking Facebook, tweeting from under the covers!
- Practice relaxation techniques, such as belly breathing.
- Dab lavender oil on your wrists or your pillow.
- Drink a calming herbal tea, such as chamomile, in the evening.

Don't:

- Exercise or engage in stimulating activities just before bed. (Do exercise, though, just earlier in the day!)
- Watch TV or use electronic devices in bed.
- Nap for more than forty-five minutes in the daytime, or after 3 P.M.
- Go to bed too hungry or too full.
- Drink too much water before bed.
- Drink alcohol or caffeine within four hours of going to bed.

- Eat heavy, spicy, or sugary foods within four hours of going to bed.
- Use the bed as an office, workroom, or recreation room.

HABIT HOMEWORK

Improve Your Sleep Hygiene

With the sleep hygiene do and don't lists from above in hand, look around your bedroom and consider making some changes:

- If you have a television in your room and have another place for it in your home, try moving it for just a week to start. Doing this will force a different routine for you at night—and that might be a very good thing.
- Do you use your phone as an alarm clock? If so, change your settings to no ring tone/no vibrate for incoming emails, texts, and notifications at night.
- Make sure that you have decent shades/window coverings so that your room doesn't get a glow from streetlights or passing headlights.

Try to Meditate

Remember that we're not talking about becoming a meditation master here. You don't have to sit cross-legged for an hour at a time to get the benefits of this ancient

YOUR PILLOW, YOUR MATTRESS, YOUR DREAMS

We all have our favorite sleeping positions, but our position of choice is more likely to be a result of unconscious habit than good sleep hygiene. It also might have something to do with how old and saggy your mattress is! Do yourself a favor and invest in a decent one—any money you spend will pay off in better zzz's!

Let's review what the experts say about how we can best position ourselves to increase our chances of drifting off to the Land of Nod.

First Choice: Sleeping on Your Back

Sleeping on your back comes in as the number one choice for a good night's rest. Back sleeping allows for a neutral position of your head and spine, so it is considered to be a good position for preventing neck and back pain. It can also help reduce acid reflux if your head is slightly elevated and your stomach is below your esophagus. But snorers beware! Sleeping on your back can exacerbate snoring and sleep apnea problems.

Second Choice: Sleeping on Your Side

If sleeping on your back doesn't work for you, try sleeping on your side. Side sleeping comes in as a close second and can provide a good position for your neck and back if you use sufficient pillow support. The pillow under your head needs to be thick enough to support your head and neck in a neutral position. You can also place a pillow between your knees and a rolled towel under your waist to support your pelvis, if you have back issues. Side sleeping can also help reduce snoring and is the position of choice during pregnancy.

To Avoid: The Fetal Position

Although curling up in the fetal position after a long day can definitely feel gratifying in the short term, consider the effects it has on your body and your sleep patterns. Spending the night with your knees pulled up high and your chin tucked into your chest will aggravate back and neck issues and can make you feel achy in the morning, especially if you suffer from arthritis. This position also compresses the belly and restricts your breathing. If you find yourself curled up, try straightening out your spine a bit and supporting your head, and see if you notice the difference.

Worst Offender: Sleeping on Your Stomach

Sleeping on your stomach is the least desirable position for a good night's sleep. It is difficult to maintain a neutral position for your head and your spine when you are sleeping on your front. If you are a front sleeper, you most likely have your head turned to one side for hours at a time, and this can lead to neck issues and back tension. You also probably sleep with one or both of your arms underneath you, which can cause sore shoulders and numbness and tingling in your arms. The one thing that sleeping on your stomach can help is snoring! So, snorers, if you do not have any back and neck issues, feel free to try it. Just make sure you use a thin pillow, or no pillow at all, to minimize the pressure on your neck and back.

practice. Think small. Try meditating for the time it takes to get to your stop on the bus or subway. If you're someone who worries about losing track of time, don't: set your phone or watch alarm to interrupt your meditation after a short period of time. You can then give yourself over to the meditation and not worry about being late for what's next on your schedule.

Try Belly Breathing

How can you *not* try this? It's so easy and it's so relaxing. Try it tonight when you get in bed.

Learn a Little Yoga

Here are the six poses you need to try. Some of these will probably look to you like good old-fashioned stretching—I'm not asking you to tie yourself up in knots or stand on your head!

You can do these any time of the day, but you'll find them most effective . . . at bedtime!

1. *Legs Up the Wall Pose/Viparita Karani*

Clear some wall/floor space in your house. (It's worth it, I promise!) Lie down on the floor, curled up on one side in the fetal position, with your bottom close to the wall. Roll slowly onto your back and straighten your legs up the wall. If it is difficult for you to straighten your legs comfortably, wriggle back a little so your butt isn't flush to the wall, or put a folded blanket or cushion under your butt to elevate your hips. Rest an eye pillow or small towel on your eyes, and gently deepen your breath. Stay for five to fifteen minutes. When you are ready to come out, draw your knees down to your chest and roll slowly onto one side.

Alternate: If having your legs up the wall is not comfort-able, or if the wall space isn't happening, you can lie on your back on the floor and rest your calves on the seat of a chair, with your hips and knees at a right angle.

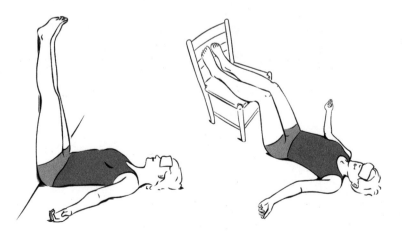

2. *Child's Pose/Balasana*

Kneel on the floor with your big toes touching and sit on your heels. Separate your knees to about hip width apart, or a little wider, and fold forward so that your torso is resting in between your thighs and your forehead is resting on the floor. Relax your arms in a comfortable position, either in front of you or at your sides. With each inhalation, allow the back of your torso to gently expand. With each exhalation, allow your forehead and pelvis to feel a little heavier. If you are uncomfortable, try placing a folded blanket or cushion under your forehead to elevate your head. Stay for several deep breaths.

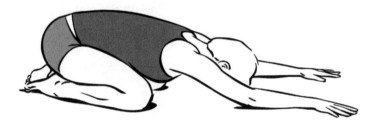

3. *Reclining Knee to Chest/Apanasana*

Lie down on the floor (or in bed) and hug both of your knees into your chest. Hold your right knee with both hands and extend your left leg straight along the floor. Hold the position for three to five deep breaths and observe your body sensations. Switch sides.

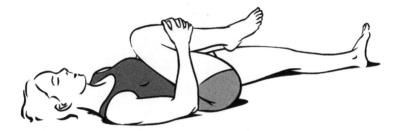

4. *Reclining Twist/Supta Matsyendrasana*

Lie down on the floor (or in bed) and hug both of your knees into your chest. Stretch out your arms to each side, resting them on the floor at the level of your shoulders. Slowly lower your bent knees all the way over to the left, and turn your head to the right. Allow your right shoulder to melt down toward the floor. Let your inhalations gently expand your ribs, and let your exhalations relax you into the twist. If your back needs support, place a pillow between your knees. If you want more stretch, place your left hand on top of your right thigh to add a little weight. Stay in the position for at least three to five breaths and observe your body sensations. Switch sides.

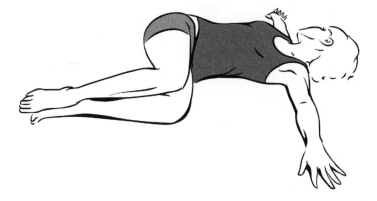

5. *Reclining Butterfly Pose/Supta Baddha Konasana*

Lie down on the floor (or in bed) with your knees bent and your feet flat on the floor. Place your feet together and allow your knees to gently drop open, with the soles of your feet touching each other. If it is difficult for you to relax your inner thighs in this position, place a pillow under each thigh so that your legs are fully supported. Rest an eye pillow or small towel on your eyes, and place your palms on your belly, just below your navel. Deepen your breath and focus on allowing your belly to gently rise up into your hands as you inhale, and soften back toward the floor as you exhale. Stay for one to five minutes.

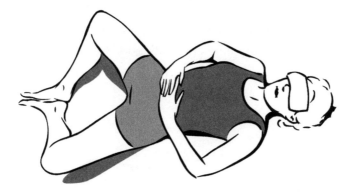

6. *Final Relaxation Pose/Corpse Pose/Savasana*

In this final relaxation pose, it is time to seriously flex your "letting go" muscle. The ancient yogis called this the most advanced yoga pose of all, as it requires complete surrender on every level. I call it the burpee of your relaxation!

Lie flat on your back on the floor (or in bed) with your limbs in a relaxed, symmetrical position. You can place a pillow under your head and/or a pillow under your knees, if that makes you more comfortable. Start to gradually relax all of your muscles, from your feet all the way up to your head. As you sense the physical tension draining out of your body, notice the back of your body becoming heavier and heavier. Let your face feel soft. Let your breath be natural. Let your thoughts come and go, like clouds floating across the sky. Remember, you are practicing letting go on every level. And, like anything else that's good for us, it does take practice! Stay for at least three minutes, or for as long as you like.

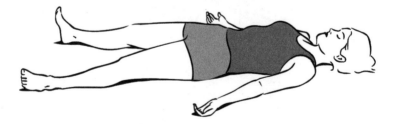

eight

HABIT 6:
DRESS FOR THIN

magine you're standing in front of your closet in a towel, post-shower. What to wear, what to wear? It's a weekday and so you're getting dressed for work. The company culture is casual and you don't work at a place that gives you a uniform. You can pretty much wear what you want, but you're feeling fat, like your usual bloated, overweight self, so you can immediately narrow things down to a few frequently worn options:

If you're a woman, those might be:

- Black elastic-waistband pants (size XL) and a loose-fitting blouse.
- Dark gray leggings (also elastic waistband, size L) and an oversized tunic-like top.

- A stretchy black pencil skirt that pinches around the waist after an hour (size M), and the same blouse from outfit 1.
- The size 12 jeans you bought when you were thinner, a loose white T-shirt, and a boxy dark blue blazer that covers your butt.

Given these choices, I'm guessing your thought process might go something like this:

Well, option 1 could be accessorized with a chunky bracelet and necklace to draw attention away from the "fat pants." Same goes for outfit 2.

That skirt is tempting—it is a medium, after all (note to self: shop more at that store because their sizing is fab!), but wearing it reminds me of my waist all day long, which is a bummer.

The jeans really aren't an option at all—getting into them is difficult, wearing them is hell, and they've been gathering dust for months—but I always put them in the running because there is a certain satisfaction to wearing size 12, no matter how uncomfortable.

All things being equal, I'll go with outfit 2 because it's comfortable without being totally sloppy. The fact that the pants are large and not XL is a bonus; getting into the medium skirt but being totally aware of the pinch at the waist all day doesn't feel worth it.

Going out tonight? Maybe, just maybe, you'll wedge yourself into those jeans since you can always unbutton them under the cover of darkness at the restaurant! Then again, add some sparkly jewelry to outfits 1 or 2 and you'll

Have you heard the argument that you should dress for the job you want, not the job you have? Reason being, other people will see you as someone who should be in charge if you dress like someone who is. Well, the same kind of psychology works on *yourself* as well as others. And when it comes to weight, the person you are trying to manipulate is *you*.

be a whole lot more comfortable at the table. Yeah, you're probably going to go with the "fat pants" for going out, too.

Work at home or not going out tonight? Break out the yoga pants and hoodie!

If you're a guy, your options aren't too dissimilar, except for the skirt and leggings. You've probably got some "Big and Tall" khaki pants (maybe they're even elastic waistband), some broken-in and baggy "fat" jeans, and some newer pants that are stiff and require a belt. For tops you've probably got a lot of T-shirts, sweaters, sweatshirts, and button-downs that you never tuck in. You have a sport coat or blazer that you keep buttoned over your beer belly. On weekends you break out your sweats—ah, comfortable at last!

There's certainly a lot to be said for having a couple of comfortable "go-to" outfits that save you time in the morning. But knowing what I do about the psychology of self-care and how it relates to weight, it shouldn't surprise you to hear that in this chapter I'm going to push you to break out of your go-to mold and make more of an effort with your appearance. Saving time in the morning is one thing, but giving up is another. We're going to have none of that from now on!

You might argue that skinny people take more care with their clothes and appearance because they have a more enviable figure to "show off," but I'm not having any of that either. I am here to tell you what I know to be true: "dressing the part" contributes to *being that person.*

YOUR BRAIN ON COMFORT AND SIZE

Mark Twain said, "The clothes make the man." In other words, either people will judge you by what you wear (which you knew already) or you can make statements about yourself through what you wear. And I'm not talking about making *fashion* statements! I'm talking about how the care you take with your appearance communicates a whole lot about your emotional state (to others) and will even *change* your emotional state (for yourself).

A study at the University of Hertfordshire a few years ago studied whether there is a link between your mood and what you choose to put on. Professor Karen Pine asked one hundred women what they choose to wear when they are depressed. Half of them said jeans. Fifty-seven percent said that they would wear a baggy top when depressed; only 2 percent said they'd wear baggy tops when happy. They also reported that they were ten times more likely to put on a favorite dress when happy (62 percent) than when they were depressed (6 percent).

Ultimately, Pine's study found that there really is something called "happy clothes." What are they? Clothing that is well-cut, figure-enhancing, and brightly colored. "Exactly the qualities jeans lack," she noted.

Another researcher, Professor Tammy Kinley at the University of North Texas, looked at this from a slightly different perspective: she wanted to see if there is a correlation between clothing *size* and self-esteem. Kinley's idea was that the very act of fitting into a smaller or larger than expected garment would affect a person's self-esteem. To test this, she recruited 149 normal-weight women and asked each to complete a questionnaire that established a baseline measure for self-esteem and body image, the size pants they buy most often, and other information about where they lived and what they did for a living. She then divided this group in two. One group would try on a brand of pants that would fit in a smaller than expected size; the other group would try on a brand of pants that would fit in a larger than expected size. Kinley later questioned the subjects about their experience and the results are probably no surprise to you: the women who tried on pants in a smaller than expected size were psyched. Anyone who did not fit into the pants they were given were sorely disappointed.

Clothing manufacturers understand the psychology at play here. They know you are likely to buy something that's in a size you don't usually fit into (sometimes even if it's more expensive). They know that you are actually more likely to buy that smaller-sized something *just because of the smaller size,* even if you don't really need it or weren't shopping for clothes in the first place. And they know that given the choice, you'll probably come back to their store because you like seeing a smaller size on the tag in your closet! So, they fudge the sizing to flatter you, to get you to come back, to get you to buy more of their "Mediums." There's even an industry term for the practice: *vanity sizing*!

You know you're guilty of vanity size shopping. Even if you know what they're up to, you chase that smaller size anyway, right? Buy the clothes with the label you like if you really like the look and feel better or if it's more reasonably priced, but don't fool yourself into thinking you've dropped a whole dress size just by walking across the street from a boutique dress shop (where sizes tend to be accurate or even smaller than normal) to a big box store (where they tend to size things larger, to make you feel smaller!)

THE BENEFITS OF TOO TIGHT

Smaller *seeming* (i.e., labeled) clothes may boost your self-esteem, but I'm guessing that *truly* smaller clothes don't, no matter how "happy" they are otherwise (colorful, nicely cut, etc.). They pinch and they press, constantly reminding you that you have weight to lose. Their bright colors and tailored lines call attention to parts of your body you'd rather hide, right?

But it turns out that having a constant physical reminder of your weight is *exactly* the thing you need. Thin and healthy people take their cues from how their clothes fit!

In the early 1980s, John Garrow, considered the dean of

obesity studies in England, got an idea for an experiment that might measure what I call "the tight clothes effect." For several years, Garrow had witnessed the rise of what, to our millennial eyes, might seem pretty barbaric: the practice of jaw wiring to help people lose weight. (I wonder what they might have thought of gastric bypass back then!) The practice, though painful and hard to endure, often worked—for a while. But when patients got their jaws unwired, they regained the weight.

Garrow pondered the situation and could see that the jaw wiring gave an obvious physical reminder and signal to eat less. He wondered what other physical signals would give the average person that same message. He decided to test something a lot less radical than jaw wiring: a waist band. Unlike today's invasive lap band procedure, Garrow's band simply wrapped around the person's waist (under their clothes, but not under their skin!). It was just tight enough to leave a white—but not red—mark when removed. It was like a slightly uncomfortable belt. After their experience with jaw wiring, half his test subjects got the band; half did not.

What happened? As Garrow wrote, the results were "a striking difference between the two groups in the weight change." In the control group, the ones who didn't get the band, weight regain commenced unchecked—by about three pounds a month. In the banded group there was no gain; the effect seemed to be a lasting one. At five months the control group had continued to regain; the banded group had regained nothing.

WARDROBE WELLNESS

Wear a Belt

Just like pants or a skirt that fits snugly around the waist, a belt is a natural gauge of how much you've eaten on a given day. If you have to loosen your belt, you know you need to push back from the table!

Keep the Stretchy Material for Your Workouts

Spandex adds stretchiness (and comfort) to clothing, but think of it this way: it also adds *give*. Wearing something with give makes it really hard to keep tabs on whether you're expanding or getting thinner.

Consider Your Shoes

The one place that pinch and discomfort isn't productive is in your feet. You don't need an excuse not to take the stairs at work or skip your evening walk! That said, wearing dress shoes (i.e., not schlumpy slip-ons) that don't hurt can make you walk the walk a little taller and more self-assuredly.

It's All About the Base

A newscaster once told me that she wears a sports bra under her professional clothes most days. Having that awkward-to-put-on base layer already in place makes it one step easier to go out for a run after work.

Garrow believed that the band helped overweight people obtain a "cognitive threshold," a kind of psychological limit to their eating. The "banding effect" seemed to continue even after the band was removed. As Garrow wrote: "It was noticeable that those patients who maintained weight loss *were those who bought new clothes that fitted at their reduced weight and warned them when their weight increased.*" They, and their tummies, had gotten the message!

In other words, while elastic waistbands and big shirts are comfortable, a little discomfort may be the reminder/ motivation you need to stick to your if/then contingency plans and make healthier food choices every day. So you should opt for that pencil skirt that pinches a little after all!

Ask my friend Amanda (from Chapter 4) how she knows when to stop eating, and she'll tell you, "It's about the pants! My clothes are one of the most important things that keep me on track. If they are tight, they remind me I'm getting fat, that I should pay attention. If they fit me well, I feel good about myself. My day is better!" Exactly!

SHOULD IT STAY OR SHOULD IT GO?

As much as I want your clothes to remind you that you need to watch what you're putting in your mouth or you need to move a little more, I don't want them to *make you feel bad.* There's a very big difference!

Clothes that are slightly snug but that once made you feel terrific have the potential—through the gentle reminder of their snugness—to make you feel terrific again one day soon. They are what I would call aspirational—they help guide you toward healthy choices.

Clothes that are too tight—that haven't really fit you in

years—well, those clothes might just sit in your closet and mock you. And they'll sap you of your emerging confidence. They'll contribute to the automatic and irrational thoughts you're trying to override with Habit 2. They'll make you feel bad about yourself every time you glimpse them. Feeling bad about yourself is *not* productive.

A recent survey by the makers of Slimfast revealed that more than two-thirds of women have fourteen items of clothing hanging in their closet that no longer fit, and they say they hold on to them in the hopes that they'll someday be able to wear them again. The thing is, there's a blurry line between a rational hope like that and an irrational attachment to clothing that maybe never fit well or suited you to begin with! You're going to have to get tough with yourself and figure out the difference.

I'm sure you've heard the rule that if you haven't worn something in a year, you should get rid of it. I actually have a slightly less rigid way of assessing what's in your closet: I want you to forget about *how long* something in your closet has been untouched and instead consider *why* it's still there. If it's there for a good reason, I don't care how long it's been on the hanger!

You'll need to come back to this self-assessment in the Habit Homework, but for now here's how to make the judgment call:

Did you wear this item of clothing for some special and memorable event, an event you don't ever want to forget? A prom or bridesmaid dress? Your wedding tux? The jeans you wore the summer you learned to drive? If the event that was memorable has nothing to do with the *size* you were when it happened, then fine, keep the clothing as a memento, but don't obsess about getting into it again. Chances are it is *way* out of fashion anyway. Keep it for your kid's dress-up box!

Are you keeping this item of clothing because it was expensive and you're determined to get your money's worth? Get over it! The money is spent and the dress gets no wear. Maybe you should bring it to a consignment shop and try to get some of that investment back. Use the earnings to buy something that fits you well now (not baggy, not loose).

Do you have the same item of clothing in several other sizes in your closet? As in, do you have four different-sized pants of the same brand and style? Come on . . . you don't need to do this to yourself. Keep the pair that fits best and the pair that fits slightly less well at the moment. Toss or donate the two pairs that are not even close.

Are you keeping this item of clothing because you loved how it made you feel when it fit right? You just loved the fabric, the fit, the flow, the looks you got when wearing it? There are legitimate reasons to keep that piece of clothing. Something just a little too tight can keep you motivated; it can even be the piece of clothing by which you measure your progress back to your ideal weight. But here's where I do want you to invoke time as a guide. Ask yourself, *When did I last try this on?* I mean, do you try it on regularly (as a measure of your progress), or has it just been sitting there in

Other results from Slimfast's survey:

- Women keep ill-fitting items for an average of fourteen months; 15 percent say they have kept pieces that don't fit for more than two years.
- Seventy-nine percent of women frequently dread getting dressed because most of their clothes don't fit.
- If it meant they could fit into everything in their closet, 57 percent said they'd be willing to wash all the dishes by hand for a month, and more than one in ten said they'd take a pay cut.
- Eighty-three percent of women admitted to lying about their pants size more often than their age!

your closet untouched because it's nowhere near fitting? If the latter, you'd be better off getting rid of its taunting presence. When you get back to your ideal weight, you can go out and celebrate by buying something new!

And don't forget this important criterion: Is this item of clothing in your closet or in your drawers because it's super comfortable and easy to slip on every day? Hmm . . . that might not be a good thing. If the clothing in question is a dumpy pair of sweatpants or a muumuu, you should toss it or give it away because you want to be wearing clothing that does more than technically fit (a tent or a garbage bag technically fits, after all!). You want to wear clothes that make you feel good about yourself!

CULTIVATING CONFIDENCE

Clothing, as well as haircuts, cosmetics, a tan, and a fresh shave, is a personal choice. Very personal. Yet according to a study commissioned by KIA (yes, the Korean car company!), there seem to be some fairly universal choices that make people feel confident. Actually, KIA did the poll to ascertain "what makes people feel sexy" as part of a rollout of a new model of car. Since feeling sexy is one way to describe feeling confident, I think it's relevant (though what will the car companies think of next?). Confidence is what we want to cultivate here. So take a look at the KIA list, in order by the most common answers, and consider if these things would help you feel confident (sexy) too:

Women

1. A new haircut
2. A sunny day
3. Walking in heels
4. Learning a new skill
5. Booking a holiday
6. Shaved legs
7. Lipstick
8. Glowing tan
9. Little black dress
10. Designer perfume

Men

1. A sunny day
2. Freshly shaved face
3. A new suit
4. Freshly brushed teeth
5. A nice-smelling aftershave
6. Being praised at work
7. A new haircut
8. Sleeping in freshly washed sheets
9. Learning a new skill
10. Someone agreeing to go on a date

HABIT HOMEWORK

Okay, chin up . . . shoulders back. It is time to tackle your wardrobe and commit to some self-care. It might be challenging to find time to do this, but trust me, this is a *vital* part of getting and staying healthily thin. Say it after me: how we look affects how we feel, and how we feel affects what we eat. Exactly! So let's get to work and polish up your armor, so you look good and shiny out there on the battlefield!

Give Yourself a Happy Clothes Makeover

Using the above rules of thumb for assessing what's been collecting dust in your closet, you're going to inventory what's there and you're going to chuck, chuck, and chuck some more. Or donate. Just get the stuff that's cluttering your closet (and hijacking you emotionally) out of your house!

GET SOME HELP: Consider hiring someone to help you organize and sort your clothing; it would be a worthwhile investment. Or find an honest friend who you think has a good sense of style, and ask her to come over and be your second set of eyes. Offer to take her out for lunch in exchange for her (brutally honest) opinions! Remember, anything that doesn't make you look *and* feel good goes on the chuck pile! When you are done, take stock of what you have left and make a list of any items you need to buy.

DONATE: Your clothes will help others, but only if you get them out the door. Getting rid of that pile of unwanted clothes is an important step on the path to staying skinny! Don't let it sit there for weeks, just in case you change your mind. You are *not* going to change your mind! Bag them up the same day, and drive them to your nearest thrift store or clothing donation box. If your brutally honest friend is with you, do it on the way to lunch!

REPLENISH: Time to go shopping. Make a list of what you need so as not to be tempted by the size 10 thing that you don't need and would never wear but want to buy because it's a size 10. Ask a stylish, honest friend to shop with you. And then be a tough judge: only buy clothes that make you look *and* feel good! Do not be swayed by vanity sizing. Pick out some key items that you need, and make sure that they fit the "happy clothes" bill—they are well-cut, figure-enhancing, and colorful. If you are not sure, put them back.

Give Yourself a Personal Makeover

So, besides fitting into those skinny jeans again, besides losing the twenty-five pounds you set out to lose last New Year's, what makes you feel good about yourself? Getting your hair cut or colored? Treating yourself to a mani/pedi? Getting a massage? Time to start a new beauty routine:

- Get a new haircut. It doesn't have to be drastic, just something that puts a spring in your step. Flick through magazines for ideas, and ask your hairdresser for advice.
- Treat yourself to a facial. If you are on a budget, treat yourself to a homemade facial. You can make an amazing low-budget face mask using food right out of your kitchen, such as avocado, honey, yogurt, and a squirt of lemon. There are endless recipes online for homemade face treats. Invite a friend over and have fun with it.
- Book yourself for a mani/pedi. If you can afford it, treat yourself to a deluxe one so that you can relax in the vibrating chair and let yourself be pampered!
- Treat yourself to a massage. It may seem like a luxury, but being comfortable in your body is an important

part of staying skinny. Tension in the body causes tension in the mind, and vice versa. And we all know where that leads . . . Most of us are more knotted up than we realize. Consider spending a day at the spa. Take a friend and enjoy a good, long soak!

SKINNY IS AS SKINNY *DOES*

Are you feeling motivated now to harness the muscle between your ears? Get started establishing your six skinny habits today. Don't wait, don't procrastinate. Set your sights on establishing one habit a week for the next six weeks, or jump in with both feet and try to do one small thing from each of the habit categories every week.

Visit www.mytrainerbob.com to let me know how you're doing. Share your accomplishments (and thoughts about how easy or hard you find the Homework) with me and with others on Facebook, Twitter, and Instagram:

- Facebook.com/MyTrainerBob
- @mytrainerbob
- Instagram.com/TrainerBob

I look forward to hearing from you!

ACKNOWLEDGMENTS

First and foremost, I have to thank my editor, Marnie Cochran, as well as the whole Random House team, for being such a delight to work with. This is my fourth book with Marnie and it has been the best experience ever. You get me. You challenge me. You understand me.

I would also like to thank my team: Greg Critser, Nicole Trinler, Richard Abate, and Brett Hansen. I've worked with this team for many years and they are always there to keep me on track and focused. I wouldn't have been able to have three #1 *New York Times* bestsellers without this team. Thank you *so much*.

I would also like to thank my CrossFit family—and by that I mean the whole CrossFit community around the world—for the dedication and loyalty they have shown me for so many years. Their solid habits with fitness and nutrition helped me to write this book. I would like to point out two Crossfitters specifically: Greg Glassman and Dave Castro. I love these two men. As founder of CrossFit, Greg Glassman has changed the landscape of fitness as we know it, and his right-hand man, Dave Castro, is a man I respect and am lucky to call friend.

Finally, my dog, Karl. My bestie and my beastie. This dog is #theshit!!

NOTES

CHAPTER 1

7 **Writing in a recent article:** V. Job, G. M. Walton, K. Bernecker, and C. S. Dweck, "Beliefs About Willpower Determine the Impact of Glucose on Self-Control," *Proceedings of the National Academy of Sciences* 110, no. 37 (Sept. 10, 2013): 14837–42.

8 **"People who didn't think willpower was limited":** Brooke Donald, "Willpower Is in Your Mind, not in a Sugar Cube, Say Stanford Scholars," Stanford Report (Stanford News Service), August 27, 2013.

8 **"When you have a limited theory of willpower":** Ibid.

CHAPTER 2

14 **Author Charles Duhigg wrote a fascinating book:** Charles Duhigg, *The Power of Habit* (New York: Random House, 2012), 3–30.

CHAPTER 3

28 **In one elegant experiment:** P. M. Gollwitzer and V. Brandstetter, "Implementation Intentions and Effective Goal Pursuit," *Journal of Personality and Social Psychology* 73, no. 1 (1997): 186–99.

31 **Dr. Gollwitzer's research—in particular a recent meta review:** G. Oettingen and P. Gollwitzer, "Chapter 7: Strategies of Setting and

Implementing Goals," in *Social Psychological Foundations of Clinical Psychology,* ed. J. E. Maddux and J. P. Tangney (New York: Guilford Press, 2010), 11735. http://www.psych.nyu.edu/gollwitzer /OettingenGollwitzer.pdf.

32 **Now meet Heidi Grant Halvorson:** For the best single source of Halvorson and her work, see www.heidigranthalvorson.com; see also H. Halvorson, *Focus* (New York: Penguin/Plume, 2013).

37 **"I was single, unhappy, and fat":** S. Flanary, interview by Greg Critser, August 6, 2014.

CHAPTER 4

46 **But one day, he had a profound insight:** Beck's complete account can be found at his website, www.beckinstituteblog.org/2007/02/.

49 **Eventually, he coined the term "cognitive distortion":** For the best two sources on cognitive distortion, see A. Beck, *Cognitive Therapies and Emotional Disorders* (New York: New American Library, 1975); and D. Burns, *Feeling Good: The New Mood Therapy* (New York: New American Library, 1980).

50 **In 2010, researchers at England's Aston University:** O. Longe et al., "Having a Word with Yourself," *Neuroimage* 49, no. 2 (January 15): 1849–56.

63 **Furthermore, she felt like she was "living in a snow globe":** A. Arlauskas, interview by Greg Critser, May 5, 2014.

CHAPTER 5

71 **In 2007, a group of Harvard researchers:** N. Christakis and N. Fowler, "The Spread of Obesity in a Large Social Network over 32 Years," *New England Journal of Medicine* 357, no. 4 (July 27, 2007): 370–79.

73 **As he recounted later:** D. Cahill, interview by Greg Critser, June 17, 2014.

75 **Or, as he put it:** M. Kruger, interview by Greg Critser, May 5, 2014.

79 **He brought sixty students into his lab/cafe:** B. Wansink, J. E. Painter, and J. North, "Bottomless Bowls: Why Visual Cues of Portion Sizes May Influence Intake," *Obesity Research* 13, no. 1 (January 2005): 93–100; and B. Wansink and K. van Ittersum, "Short, Wide Glasses Induce Us to Over-Pour Despite Serving Experience," *Journal of Consumer Research* 30 (December 2003): 455–64. Also see Wansink's

seminal book on environmental influences on eating: B. Wansink, *Mindless Eating: Why We Eat More Than We Think* (New York: Bantam Books, 2006).

81 **"If there's a box of cookies":** A. Kingston, "The Interview: Brian Wansink on Why We Eat What We Eat," *Maclean's,* September 20, 2014; online at www.macleans.ca/society/the-interview-brian-wansink-on-food-and-eating/.

81 **"It could be that sitting next to a window cues the mind":** Ibid.

82 **"I needed that feeling of changing":** D. Cahill, interview by Greg Critser, June 17, 2014.

CHAPTER 6

94 **In 2012, a group of researchers at Emory University:** B. Hanna-Pladdy and B. Gajewski, "Recent and Past Musical Activity Predicts Cognitive Aging Variability: Direct Comparison with General Lifestyle Activities," *Frontiers in Human Neuroscience* 6 (July 19, 2012): 198.

96 **In a 2008 report, researchers reported the results of another scanning study:** C. Sampaio-Baptista et al., "Gray Matter Volume Is Associated with Rate of Subsequent Skill Learning After a Long Term Training Intervention," *Neuroimage* 96 (August 1, 2014): 158–66.

97 **Participants in a community study of quilters:** E. L. Burt and J. Atkinson, "The Relationship Between Quilting and Well-Being," *Journal of Public Health* 34, no. 1 (March 2012): 54–59.

98 **Danny Cahill, the reengineering mastermind:** D. Cahill, interview with Greg Critser, June 15, 2014; also personal email communication with Greg Critser, November 6, 2014.

CHAPTER 7

108 **A recent study at the University of California, Berkeley:** S. M. Greer, A. N. Goldstein, and M. P. Walker, "The Impact of Sleep Deprivation on Food Desire in the Human Brain," *Nature Communications* 4 (August 6, 2013): 2259.

109 **Sleep researchers from the University of Colorado:** R. Markwalda et al., "Impact of Insufficient Sleep on Total Daily Energy Expenditure," *Proceedings of the National Academy of Sciences* 110, no. 14 (March 11, 2013), 5695–700.

109 **Other studies on the metabolic consequences:** F. Garcia-Garcia et al., "Ghrelin and Its Interactions with Growth Hormone, Leptin and Orexins: Implications for the Sleep-Wake Cycle and Metabolism," *Sleep Medicine Reviews* 18, no. 1 (February 2014): 89–97.

110 **Some studies have shown an increase in cortisol levels:** K. Spiegel, R. Leproult, and E. Van Cauter, "Impact of Sleep Debt on Metabolic and Endocrine Function," *Lancet* 354 (1999): 1435–39. See also R. Leproult, G. Copinschi, O. Buxton, and E. Van Cauter, "Sleep Loss Results in an Elevation of Cortisol Levels the Next Evening," *Sleep* 20, no. 10 (October 1997): 865–70; and Eun Yeon Ju, Cindy W. Yoon, Dae Lim Koo, Daeyoung Kim, and Seung Bong Hong, "Adverse Effects of 24 Hours of Sleep Deprivation on Cognition and Stress Hormones," *Journal of Clinical Neurology* 8, no. 2 (June 2012): 146–50.

110 **A small study carried out at the University of Chicago:** J. L. Broussard et al., "Impaired Insulin Signaling in Human Adipocytes After Experimental Sleep Restriction," *Annals of Internal Medicine* 157, no. 8 (October 16, 2012): 549–57.

113 **He wrote a bestselling book by the same name in 1975:** H. Benson, *The Relaxation Response*, reissue edition (New York: HarperTorch, 2000).

114 **An interesting experiment was conducted at the University of Utah:** W. R. Marchand, "Neural Mechanisms of Mindfulness Meditation: Evidence from Neuroimaging Studies," *World Journal of Radiology* 6, no. 7 (July 28, 2014): 471–79. Also, for an outstanding introduction to mindfulness meditation, see http://counselingcenter.utah .edu/services/mindfulness.php.

116 **"In conclusion, our results demonstrate":** H. Woelk and S. Schläfke, "A Multi-Center, Double-Blind, Randomised Study of the Lavender Oil Preparation Silexan in Comparison to Lorazepam for Generalized Anxiety Disorder," *Phytomedicine* 17, no. 2 (February 2010): 94–99.

117 **In 2006, a group of researchers at the University of Duisburg-Essen:** A. Michalsen et al., "Rapid Stress Reduction and Anxiolysis Among Distressed Women as a Consequence of a Three-Month Intensive Yoga Program," *Medical Science Monitor* 11, no. 12 (December 2005): 555–61.

CHAPTER 8

134 **A study at the University of Hertfordshire:** B. Fletcher and K. Pine, *FLEX: Do Something Different: How to Use the Other 9/10ths of Your Personality* (Hertfordshire, UK: University of Hertfordshire Press, 2012). For the best summary of Pine's work. see http://karenpine .com/wp-content/uploads/2012/03/PR-Happiness-its-not-in-the -jeans.pdf.

135 **Another researcher, Professor Tammy Kinley:** T. R. Kinley, "The Effect of Clothing Size on Self-Esteem and Body Image," *Family & Consumer Science* 38, no. 3 (March 2010): 317–32.

136 **In the early 1980s, John Garrow:** J. S. Garrow and G. T. Gardiner, "Maintenance of Weight Loss in Obese Patients After Jaw Wiring," *British Medical Journal* (Clinical Research Edition) 282, no. 6267 (March 14, 1981): 858–60.

139 **As Garrow wrote: "It was noticeable":** Ibid., 860.

140 **A recent survey by the makers of Slimfast:** "Slimfast Reveals 'Locked Closet Syndrome' and Other Wardrobe Hang-Ups," Slimfast website, press release, May 12, 2014, www.unileverusa.com/media-center /pressreleases/2014/SlimfastInvitesWomenToUnlockYourClosetWith 14-DaySlimdown.aspx.

143 **Yet according to a study commissioned by KIA:** M. Davies, "Here's What Makes a Woman Feel Sexy, Apparently," Jezebel.com, May 30, 2014, http://jezebel.com/heres-what-makes-a-woman-feel -sexy-apparently-1583941255.

INDEX

action-thought-action cycles, xiii–xiv
alcohol use, 105, 120
anxiety
  hatha yoga, 117–18
  lavender oil, 116, 120
  shame, 50–51
  See also relaxation
Apanasana, 127
arcuate fasciculus, 95–96
Arlauskas, Amanda, 63–65
asanas, 115, 124–30
assumptions, 4–9
Ativan, 116
atta-boy "rule," 60
attitudes, 4–9
automatic responses. *See* default
  responses

back sleeping, 122
bad filters, 49–51

Balasana, 126
basal ganglia, 13, 114
base layers, 138
Beck, Aaron, 46–49
bedtime routines, 118–20
behaviors, xv
  irrational behaviors, 26–27,
    43–60
  replacement behaviors, 18–21, 27
  See also habit-making
belly breathing, 113, 118–19, 120,
  124
belts, 138
beneficial hormones, 106
Benson, Herbert, 113
benzodiazepines, 116
biases, 4–9
The Biggest Loser, xi, 63–65, 73–74
black-and-white thinking, 51–52
blame-gaming, 55–56

blood sugar, 12–13
boredom, xiv, 90–92, 94
brain functions, 12–21
　arcuate fasciculus, 95–96
　basal ganglia, 13, 114
　clothing and emotional states,
　　134–36
　default responses, 26–27, 43–60
　fuel consumption, 12–13
　if/then options, 30–33
　learning and mental agility,
　　92–99
　making memories, 14–18,
　　92–93
　medial temporal lobe, 13
　meditation, 114–15, 121, 124
　REM sleep, 107
　replacement behaviors, 18–21, 27
　shame, 50–51
　sleep, 106
breathing exercises, 115
Buddhism, 113–15
buffets, 83
built environments, 68–69, 76–83
　food-related decisions, 76–81
　homework, 85–88
　obese-o-genic theory, 78–80
　reengineering of, 82–83
　supermarkets, 77

caffeine, 120
Cahill, Danny, 73–75, 82, 98–99
catastrophizing, 53
challenging yourself, xiv, xvi,
　　89–101
　boredom, 90–92
　homework, 89, 99–101

learning and mental agility, 92–97
　service to others, 97–100
change delusions, 58
changing your habits, xiv, xv
　mindsets, 3–9, 11
　replacement behaviors, 18–21, 27
child's pose, 126
chronic stress, 112
chunking, 14
circadian rhythm, 104–8
clean sleep, 118–20
closet inventories, 144–46
clothing. See dressing for thinness
cognitive behavioral therapy
　　(CBT), 46–51
computer screens, 105, 120
confidence, 143–44
conscious mental pushbacks. See
　　pushing back
constipation, 112
contingency plans, 24–27
　See also if/then statements
control-ism, 54–55
cooking, 4
corpse pose, 130
cortisol levels, 110, 117
creating new behaviors. See
　　behaviors
cue-behavior-reward process,
　　14–15, 18–19

daytime rhythms, 105–6
default responses, 26–27, 43–60
　bad filters, 49–51
　black-and-white thinking, 51–52
　blame-gaming, 55–56
　catastrophizing, 53

change delusions, 58
cognitive behavioral therapy
   (CBT), 46–49
control-ism, 54–55
expecting praise, 60
fairness delusion, 55
feelings as facts, 57
global labeling, 58–59
judging yourself, 54
mind reading, 52–53
overgeneralizing, 52
perfectionism, 59–60
pushing back, 61–66
shame, 50–51
"should" lists, 56–57
delta sleep, 107
depression, 50–51
diabetes, 108, 110
dog companions, 36–37
dreaming, 107
dressing for thinness, xv–xvi,
   131–47
   belts and waistbands, 137–39
   closet inventories, 144–46
   clothing size, 135–36
   confidence, 143–44
   happy clothes, 134–35
   homework, 144–47
   personal makeovers, 146–47
   snug clothes, 136–39
   too-tight clothes, 139–42
dry mouth syndrome, 112
Duhigg, Charles, 14
Dweck, Carol, 6–9

environments, 37–38
   built environments, 68–69, 76–83

food environments, 37–38
   reengineering your environment,
      xiv, xv–xvi, 67–88
   social environments, 68–76
exercise
   if/then statements, 41–42
   workout buddies, 85

facials, 146
fairness delusion, 55
fat cells, 110
fat-shame-regain cycle, 35–37
fat traps. See built environments
feelings as facts, 57
fetal position, 123
fight-or-flight responses, 50–51,
   111–13
final relaxation pose, 130
fixed mindsets, 5–9
Flanary, Scott, 35–39
fMRIs, 93
food, 4
   brain fuel, 12–13
   calorie content, 87
   sleep hygiene, 120–21
food environments, 37–38, 76–81
   See also social environments
Framingham Heart Study, 71–72
front sleeping, 123
fuel, 12–13
functional MRIs, 93

Garrow, John, 136–39
generalized anxiety disorder
   (GAD), 116
ghrelin, 110
global labeling, 58–59

glucose, 12–13
goal setting, xiv–xvi, 33–34
Gollwitzer, Peter, 27–31
growth hormone, 106
growth mindsets, 5–9

habit-making
  cue-behavior-reward process,
    14–15, 18–19
  default responses, 26–27
  if/then statements, 27–42
  replacement behaviors, 18–21, 27
  See also changing your habits;
    learning
habits of mind, xiv, xv, 3–9
  See also mindsets
haircuts, 146
Halvorson, Heidi Grant, 32, 36–37
happy clothes, 134–35
Harper, Bob, 149
hatha yoga, 115–18, 124–30
heart disease, 108
hobbies, 92–101
homework
  challenging yourself, 89, 99–101
  dressing for thinness, 144–47
  if/then statements, 39–42
  pushing back, 65–66
  reengineering your environment,
    84–88
  rest, 121–30
hormones, 106, 109–10
hunger hormone, 110

if/then statements, 27–42
  exercise, 41–42
  healthy eating, 40–41

thinking positive, 35
thinking small, 33–34
immune system, 106, 108
implementation intentions, 27–31
inflating, 53
insulin, 110
intentions. *See* if/then statements
internal scripts, xiv, xv
irrational behaviors. *See* default
  responses

jaw wiring, 137
judging yourself, 54
juggling, 96

Kinley, Tammy, 135
Kruger, Mark, 75–76

lack of sleep, 108–11
lavender oil, 116, 120
learned behavior, 32–33
learning, 14–18
  cue-behavior-reward process,
    14–15, 18–19
  increasing mental agility, 93–99
  replacement behaviors,
    18–21, 27
  sticky memories, 16–17, 92–93
legs-up-the-wall pose, 125
leptin, 109–10

macro environments, 77–81
makeovers, 146–47
manicures, 146
massage, 146–47
mattresses, 122
meals, 4

medial temporal lobe, 13
meditation, 113–15, 121, 124
memories, 13–18
 chunking, 14
 cue-behavior-reward process,
  14–15, 18–19
 replacement behaviors, 18–21, 27
 sticky memories, 16–17, 92–93
 See also brain functions; habit-
  making
mental muscle, xiv, xv, 92–97
 See also brain functions; learning
mental pushbacks. *See* pushing
 back
metabolism, 109
micro environments, 77–81
mindfulness meditation, 113–15,
 121, 124
mind reading, 52–53
mindsets, 3–9, 11
 conscious mental pushbacks,
  43–44, 61–66
 willpower, 4, 6–9, 11, 26
 See also brain functions
mood
 clothing, 134–36
 depression, 50–51
motivation, 27–28
 See also willpower
musical practice, 95–96

naps, 120
nausea, 112
negative self-talk. *See* default
 responses
negative words, 35
n-REM phase sleep, 106–7

obese-o-genic theory, 78–80
obesity
 chronic stress, 112
 macro food environments,
  78–81
 sleep deprivation, 108–11
 social transmission, 71–72
outlook on life, 4–9
overgeneralizing, 52

pedicures, 146
perfectionism, 59–60
personal makeovers, 146–47
pet-companions, 36–37
phones, 105, 120, 121
Pine, Karen, 134–35
planning, xiv, xv, 23–42
 contingencies, 24–27
 default responses, 26–27
 emergencies, 24
 homework practice, 39–42
 if/then statements, 27–42
 pet companions, 36–37
 replacement behaviors, 27
 thinking positive, 35
 thinking small, 33–34
positive words, 35
The Power of Habit (Duhigg), 14
praise, 60
pranayama, 115
psychological habits, xiv, xv
pushing back, xiv, xv, 43–66
 cognitive behavioral therapy
  (CBT), 46–49
 default responses, 43–60
 homework, 65–66
 rational self-reassurance, 61–66

quilting, 96–97

rapid-eye-movement (REM) sleep, 107
rational self-interest, 78–81
rational self-reassurance, 50–51, 61–66
recipes, 4
reclining butterfly pose, 129
reclining knee to chest pose, 127
reclining twist pose, 128
reengineering your environment, xiv–xvi, 67–88
  built environments, 68–69, 76–83
  homework, 84–88
  social environments, 68–76
relationships. *See* social environments
relaxation, 94, 112–30
  belly breathing, 113, 118–19, 120, 124
  mindfulness meditation, 113–15, 121, 124
  relaxation response, 112–13
  yoga, 113, 115–18, 124–30
  See also rest
REM sleep, 107
replacement behaviors, 18–21, 27
rest, xv, xvi, 103–30
  homework, 121–30
  relaxation, 94, 112–30
  sleep, 103–8
  sleep deprivation, 108–11
  stress response, 111–13
restaurant meals
  buffets, 83
  seating, 81

satiety hormone, 109–10
Savasana, 130
self-control, 4, 6–9
self-reassurance, 50–51, 61–66
semiboredom, 92
service to others, 97–100
serving size, 81
shame, 50–51
shoes, 138
shopping routines, 84–85
"should" lists, 56–57
side sleeping, 122–23
silexan, 116
six habits of skinny, xiii–xvi, 149, 173
  challenging yourself, xiv, xvi, 89–101
  dressing for thinness, xv–xvi, 131–47
  planning, xiv–xv, 23–42
  pushing back, xiv–xv, 43–66
  reengineering your environment, xiv–xvi, 67–88
  rest, xv–xvi, 103–30
Skinny Meals (Harper), 4
The Skinny Rules (Harper), xi–xii, 4, 67, 103
sleep, 103–11
  bedtime routines, 118–20
  biology of fat cells, 110
  circadian rhythm, 104–5
  cortisol levels, 110, 117
  daytime activities, 105–6
  deprivation, 108–11
  hormone levels, 106, 109–10
  metabolism and eating habits, 109

positions, 122–23
sleep cycles, 106–8
sleep-related disease, 108
sleep apnea, 122
sleep hygiene, 118–23
sleeping pills, 104
sleep-wake cycles, 104–8
Slimfast, 140
slip-shame-binge cycle, xii–xiv, 61–63
snoring, 122–23
snug clothes, 136–39
social environments, 68–76
    homework, 84–85
    reengineering of, 73–76
    transmission of obesity, 71–72
Soup Bowl Study, 79–80
spandex, 138
splurges, 25
sticky memories, 16–17, 92–93
stomach sleeping, 123
stress levels, 110
    chronic stress, 112
    shallow breathing, 118
    yoga, 117–18
stress response, 50–51, 111–13
supermarkets, 77, 84–85
supporting your goals, xiv–xvi

Supta Baddha Konasana, 129
Supta Matsyendrasana, 128

television, 120, 121
testosterone, 106
thinking positive, 35
thinking small, 33–34
"tight clothes effect," 137–39
too-tight clothes, 139–42
toxic boredom, 90–92, 94
Twain, Mark, 134
twenty rules for getting thin, xi–xii, 67, 175

vanity sizing, 136
Viparita Karani, 125

waistbands, 137–39
Wansink, Brian, 78–81, 83, 85
wardrobe choices. *See* dressing for thinness
water, 103, 120
willpower, 4, 6–9, 11, 25–26
workout buddies, 85
www.mytrainerbob.com, 149

yoga, 113, 115–18, 124–30

ABOUT THE AUTHORS

BOB HARPER is a world-renowned fitness trainer and the longest-reigning star of the NBC reality series *The Biggest Loser*, which finished its sixteenth season in 2015. He has released several popular fitness DVDs and is the author of the number one *New York Times* bestselling books *The Skinny Rules, Jumpstart to Skinny,* and *Skinny Meals.* Harper lives in Los Angeles with his dog, Karl.

www.mytrainerbob.com
Facebook.com/mytrainerbob
@mytrainerbob

GREG CRITSER is a longtime science and medical journalist. The author of the international bestseller *Fat Land: How Americans Became the Fattest People in the World,* he lives in Pasadena, California.

ABOUT THE TYPE

THIS BOOK was set in Granjon, a modern recutting of a typeface produced under the direction of George W. Jones, who based Granjon's design upon the letter forms of Claude Garamond (1480–1561). The name was given to the typeface as a tribute to the typographic designer Robert Granjon.

THE SKINNY HABITS RECAP

1. **Make Contingency Plans:** To avoid unhealthy eating, encourage exercise, resist temptation, and guard against that first slip, create your own internal scripts for dealing with difficult situations.

2. **Consciously Push Back:** Notice your automatic thoughts and pinpoint which kind of "distorted" thinking you're engaging in. Develop the mental muscle to deal with setbacks (aka the cascading shame from inevitable slipups).

3. **Reengineer Your Environment:** Rig your home, office, and social life to accentuate the people, places, and things that support your goals, and deemphasize (or eliminate) those that don't.

4. **Challenge Yourself:** Boredom is the gateway to overeating and sitting around like a lump on your couch. Keep your mind engaged and excited about something other than the monotony of your daily responsibilities.

5. **Rest for Success:** You can be engaged, excited, focused, and energized only if you are rested. Protect your sleep, and find time for even small moments of relaxation.

6. **Dress for Thin:** Don't hide behind your baggy clothes, however comfortable they are! Reap the psychological and physiological benefits of clothes that really fit (or that remind you of the weight you want to lose).

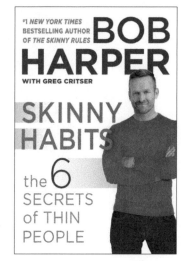

#1 NEW YORK TIMES
BESTSELLING AUTHOR
OF THE SKINNY RULES **BOB HARPER**

WITH GREG CRITSER

SKINNY HABITS

the 6 SECRETS of THIN PEOPLE

(cut this page out and post where you'll see it daily)

THE SKINNY RULES RECAP

RULE 1: Drink a Large Glass of Water Before Every Meal— No Excuses!

RULE 2: Don't Drink Your Calories

RULE 3: Eat Protein at Every Meal—or Stay Hungry and Grouchy

RULE 4: Slash Your Intake of Refined Flours and Grains

RULE 5: Eat 30 to 50 Grams of Fiber a Day

RULE 6: Eat Apples and Berries Every Single Day. Every. Single. Day!

RULE 7: No Carbs After Lunch

RULE 8: Learn to Read Food Labels So You Know What You Are Eating

RULE 9: Stop Guessing About Portion Size and Get It Right— for Good

RULE 10: No More Added Sweeteners, Including Artificial Ones

RULE 11: Get Rid of Those White Potatoes

RULE 12: Make One Day a Week Meatless

RULE 13: Get Rid of Fast Foods and Fried Foods

RULE 14: Eat a Real Breakfast

RULE 15: Make Your Own Food and Eat at Least Ten Meals a Week at Home

RULE 16: Banish High-Salt Foods

RULE 17: Eat Your Vegetables— Just Do It!

RULE 18: Go to Bed Hungry

RULE 19: Sleep Right

RULE 20: Plan One Splurge Meal a Week

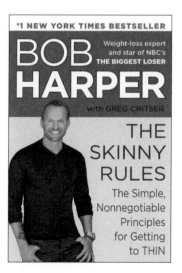

#1 NEW YORK TIMES BESTSELLER

BOB HARPER

Weight-loss expert and star of NBC's THE BIGGEST LOSER

with GREG CRITSER

THE SKINNY RULES

The Simple, Nonnegotiable Principles for Getting to THIN

(cut this page out and post where you'll see it daily)